T0386598

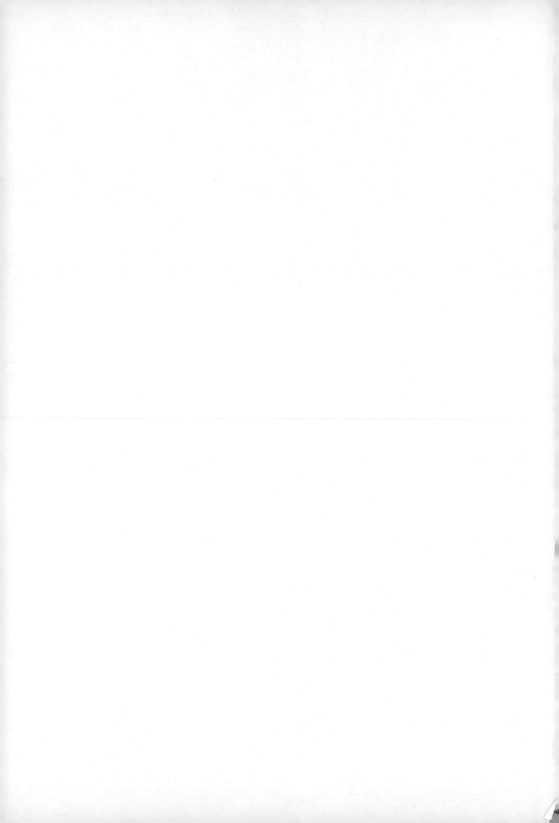

Becoming a Nurse

A hermeneutic study of the experiences of student nurses on a Project 2000 course

THERESA MITCHELL
University of the West of England

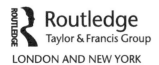

Routledge
Taylor & Francis Group

LONDON AND NEW YORK

First published 2002 by Ashgate Publishing

Reissued 2018 by Routledge
2 Park Square, Milton Park, Abingdon, Oxon OX14 4RN
711 Third Avenue, New York, NY 10017, USA

Routledge is an imprint of the Taylor & Francis Group, an informa business

Publisher's Note
The publisher has gone to great lengths to ensure the quality of this reprint but points out that some imperfections in the original copies may be apparent.

Disclaimer
The publisher has made every effort to trace copyright holders and welcomes correspondence from those they have been unable to contact.

A Library of Congress record exists under LC control number: 2001096519

ISBN 13: 978-1-138-72640-6 (hbk)
ISBN 13: 978-1-138-72637-6 (pbk)
ISBN 13: 978-1-315-19139-3 (ebk)

Contents

v

List of Figures and Tables

Figures

Tables

List of Appendices

Abstract

Becoming a nurse - a hermeneutic study of the experiences of student nurses on a Project 2000 course

The professional socialisation of students into the role of the nurse has been the focus of many research studies, the majority of which assert that individuals pass through a recognised process of 'becoming'. The purpose of this study was to explore the nature and meaning of experiences which enabled students to develop a concept of themselves as a nurse. It uses Heidegger's hermeneutic phenomenological approach to gain insight into the unique and common experiences of students.

The methodology constitutes original and creative approaches to data collection and analysis. Eight students' development and changing constructs were captured at seven data collection phases over a three year period. Focus groups with nurse tutors (N=27) and interviews with practitioners (N=15), provided contextual data against which students' stories have been portrayed.

Data were analysed using Reinharz's (1983) framework to identify common and unique experiences. The hermeneutic concepts of 'intentionality', 'thrownness', 'being-in-the-world-with-others', 'temporality' and 'active subject' illuminate the students' experiences.

The research will inform my own practice as a senior lecturer particularly in the areas of student supervision, student reflection, student development, teaching and leadership skills and in strategies to enhance student confidence when dealing with dying patients and bereaved relatives.

The research contributes to both ongoing discussions in the literature related to socialisation theories and to the qualitative methodology literature.

Preface

During the last decade, nurse education has undergone radical changes in order to meet the healthcare demands of future generations. The realisation that traditional nurse training would be inadequate to meet the various healthcare requirements resulted in the development of nurse education curricula with the intention of preparing knowledgeable, skilled practitioners. Historically, nursing has been renowned for its dependence upon the medical profession and a poorly defined, unique body of knowledge. Indeed, French (1992) proposed that in the past, pre-registration preparation for nurses was not an educational experience at all and that it produced trained practitioners who were uncritical replicators of existing nursing practice.

In May 1986 the United Kingdom Central Council (UKCC) for Nursing, Midwifery and Health Visiting published its proposals for the reform of nurse education under the title "Project 2000 - A New Preparation for Practice" (UKCC, 1986). Reforms in nurse education had repeatedly called for radical change and this policy document emphasised influential aspects such as demographic changes, emphasis upon community care rather than institutional care and a trend towards preventative health care, as opposed to a more reactionary approach to ill health.

The first colleges and schools of nursing to implement Project 2000 curricula were labelled 'demonstration districts' and these educational institutions recruited student nurses, on the Project 2000 courses, in different areas around Britain. Subsequent evaluations at various times throughout the implementation ensued, with particular reference to the effectiveness of the Courses in producing efficient, knowledgeable practitioners (Bradby and Soothill, 1993; Jowett, Walton and Payne, 1994; May, Veitch, McIntosh and Alexander, 1997; Ramprogus, 1995).

In 1992 students embarked upon the first Project 2000 course in the school where I was a nurse tutor. I had taken part in developmental meetings for the curriculum which had been planned some years before. My role as a nurse tutor meant that I was involved with Project 2000 students from the outset as a teacher of 'research awareness' and 'nursing theory/practice' modules and as an 'academic tutor' responsible for facilitating students writing their assignments. The climate at that time was tense and expectant and people were hopeful for the future but disappointed with what appeared to be a theory-biased curriculum. Many nurse tutors were unable, or not prepared, to undertake roles within the remit of Project 2000 because of the academic demands made upon them and the perception that nursing as such, had been lost within academia. This resulted in several tutors in my work area leaving nurse education posts. From a personal perspective I found the challenge exciting, stimulating and rewarding and enjoyed participating in discussions amongst my colleagues. I was also intrigued by students' stories relating to tensions in clinical practice and the strategies they would employ in order to be accepted by their qualified counterparts. However, they also expressed that they felt unprepared for practice but demonstrated an overwhelming desire to possess nurse status despite the many obstacles and distractions experienced in the educational and clinical environment. I found some of these stories alarming and became concerned about the general well-being of student nurses who were trying to gain experience within the realms of Project 2000.

The following questions evolved from my own experiences as a nurse tutor with Project 2000 student nurses:

- What perceptions do student nurses have of Project 2000 as they embark upon the Course?
- What difficulties do they encounter in clinical practice?
- What meaning do they assign to significant experiences in practice?
- Who is influential in the development of students into qualified practitioners?
- How do students' constructs of nursing develop during the three year nurse education programme?
- How do significant experiences and everyday practices influence student nurses' development during the three year nurse education programme?

This research was concerned with gaining an insight into the student nurse's lifeworld and how perceptions and significant experiences furnished nurses with meaning about being and becoming a nurse. I collected data between 1994 and 1997 whilst employed as a nurse tutor in the study area. Towards the end of the fieldwork, the College of Health became the Faculty of Health and Social Care within a University and, although my title changed to senior lecturer, my role with Project 2000 (Diploma of Higher Education in Nursing Studies) students was similar. The unique and common themes which emerged from the data have implications for nurse education and nursing practice; I also hope

to provoke discussion and inspire an enthusiasm for the research
methods and techniques I used in this study.

Acknowledgements

This study would not have been possible without the co-operation and enthusiasm of the student nurses who participated in it. My sincere thanks to Ben, Carol, Clare, Cathy, David, Marie, Paula and Sarah. Also to the tutors and practitioners who participated in the focus groups and interviews which provided data for Chapter 4.

There were many people who gave me sustained encouragement and support throughout the course of this study, but I would like to thank especially Professor Mary Fuller for her consistent, patient feedback and tolerance and Dr. Anthony Rosie, who endured this project with me for six years and always inspired me to look beyond the obvious.

Thank you to Professor Julienne Meyer, my third supervisor, who was instrumental in my success at transfer from M.Phil. to Ph.D. and to Jane Wathen who transformed my original thesis into this book.

Finally, thank you to my partner, Martin Smith for having faith in me and for providing support and understanding during my quest to meet this challenge.

Part I

Modality and Motivation

1 Introduction

The introduction is usually written last, for only then will I be sure of what the account is about.

(Woods, 1999, p21)

It may seem strange to begin with this quotation, but for me, writing the introduction signifies a point of departure - the point where my work is handed over to the reader, and ownership of it ceases to be mine alone.

The journey encountered during the last six years has taken me through rough terrain, unknown territory and has exposed me to experiences associated with the intense pleasures and frustrations of being a part-time student in addition to full-time employee. The challenge has tested my stamina, stretched my capacity to learn and jousted with my character. My strengths have been illuminated and limitations exposed.

The aim in this introductory chapter is twofold; firstly to give reasons for my choice of topic and situate my research within the associated, existing literature and secondly to introduce the structure and style of the book to the reader and indicate the format of the study.

Background to the study

During the last decade nurse education has undergone significant transformation from the old 'apprenticeship' system to a diploma level education built upon a firm theoretical base. The desired outcome of these radical changes is an independent, assertive, autonomous nurse practitioner who is capable of responding to the health care needs of the population in the future (UKCC, 1986).

Within a diploma course [initially called 'Project 2000' because of its intention to prepare nurses for the year 2000 and beyond] students embarked upon a programme of study which, at the time this research was conducted, consisted of an initial 18 month common foundation period followed by a further 18 months in the chosen branch programme of either adult general, mental health, learning disabilities or sick children's nursing. Project 2000 courses and subsequent courses derived from them contrast with the traditional nurse training model

3

which I experienced as a student nurse, where we were part of the National Health Service (NHS) workforce and were therefore employed by the NHS, received a certificate level education, learned 'on the job' and were then registered as a nurse. By contrast, Project 2000 students receive a bursary, gain a diploma in higher education and registration for their chosen branch of nursing. The Diploma course demands greater academic involvement by the students where the emphasis has been on the application of theory to practice, rather than the acquisition of practical skills in order to 'do the job' as advocated on traditional courses.

Despite the demand for higher academic performance from students, minimum entry requirements remained the same, (5 GCSEs at A, B or C grade) although each college of nursing had their own stipulation with regard to entry qualifications.

The perceptions and experiences of student nurses have been of interest to educationalists for a long time. Professional socialisation of students into the role of the nurse has provided the focus for many research studies (Bradby, 1989; Buckenham, 1998; Conway, 1993; Davis-Martin, 1990; Day, Field, Campbell and Reutter, 1995; Macleod Clark, Maben and Jones, 1996; Melia, 1981; Oleson and Whitaker, 1968; Simpson, 1979; Wilson and Startup, 1991; Wyatt, 1978). All these studies, except Macleod Clark et al. (1996) and Buckenham (1998) were concerned with the occupational socialisation of students into nursing through traditional nurse training prior to the introduction of Project 2000 curricula. Without exception, they viewed socialisation as a process whereby those being socialised acquire the attitudes and values, with the skills and behaviour patterns, that constitute the 'professional role'.

Professional socialisation is regarded as a specific aspect of adult socialisation (Goldenberg and Iwasiw, 1993) and is thought to occur through complex interactive processes which enable the professional role to be learned and the values, attitudes and goals, integral to the profession, to be internalised. For a full explanation of the complexities of adult socialisation theory, see Feldman (1976), Grbich (1990) and Mortimer and Simmons (1978).

My reading of the socialisation literature was motivated by high attrition and wastage rates for the first two Project 2000 courses in the area where this study was conducted. Only one third of all those who started the Course completed three years later and registered as nurses. As a nurse tutor I was concerned by students' stories of thwarted expectations, disillusionment and dissatisfaction with the Project 2000 course [also noted by Parker and Carlisle, 1996] and subsequently by

4

their lack of enthusiasm to continue. It seemed to me that this new, demanding and somewhat challenging phenomenon needed investigating for its impact upon individuals who wanted to be nurses.

My intention in the next section is to review pertinent socialisation studies which informed me of the overall picture in the nursing literature. It is not a review to provide background to the whole study, as I shall be introducing literature from a range of sources at appropriate points in the book.

An overview of pertinent nurse socialisation studies

Wyatt's (1978) study focused upon the theory-practice gap and student experiences in hospital settings and was reviewed because of its similarity to Melia's (1981) study conducted in 1979. Twenty-seven student nurses were interviewed in Wyatt's study either in their second or third year of training. The data were analysed using a framework suggested by Becker, Geer and Hughes (1968), which proposes three components in the acquisition of a perspective; the definition of the situation, the activities one may engage in and the criteria of judgement used in the situation. All the participants in Wyatt's study were female and comments relating to the 'remoteness' between tutors and students because of age differences imply that the students may well have been direct entrants from school. The aim was to elicit the perceptions of student nurses of their role and learning experiences on the wards, but all the student data were aggregated and analysed using descriptive statistics to determine 'good' and 'bad' features of training and the General Nursing Council syllabus. Within the analysis, there was no acknowledgement of individual development during training and no male or mature entrant perspective.

As a result of critiquing the socialisation studies of her time, Simpson (1979) is adamant that socialisation must be seen as individual change, perceived as a process or outcome or both. She supports the view that, in order to capture the essence of socialisation, examination of responses from the same individual at different points in time is essential. This enables the identification of persistent or changing dispositions or actions in response to exposure to nursing education and practice. Simpson cautions researchers against using data from different subjects at different times in a longitudinal study of socialisation and comments that snapshots are static and, even if chronologically arranged, may obscure connections which create diachronic patterns for an individual.

5

One of the findings from Simpson's study, which was completed in 1965, was that students went into nursing to help others. They were less concerned with self expression, competitive achievement or other values that would individuate them. Students were not attracted to academic courses or experiences such as contact with non-nursing students which would de-emphasise or void their status as student nurses. Insulation of student nurses from other university students is an interesting issue which has been raised by the participants in my study (Chapters 8 and 9). Simpson's large study revealed that occupational orientations are acquired; they do not simply mature.

The core contribution of Melia's (1981) classic work is an analysis of student interviews at various stages during the three year traditional training period. Her study examined the issues discussed between herself and the students and provides a snapshot of experiences from students at different stages of their course. Data for Melia's study were collected over a period of 18 months, comprising 40 hours of interviews at 8, 18 or 30 months into their training for the General Register. This means that she did not access any students undertaking mental health, learning disability or sick children's nursing. The emphasis of her study is upon ward work and hands-on care and themes emerged concerning learning and working concurrently.

Six themes emerged from Melia's data: "Learning and working" referred to those experiences associated with the theory-practice gap; "Getting the work done" included descriptions of nursing work and the management styles employed on hospital wards; "Learning the rules" evolved through students' experiences of on-the-job training and expectations of them on the wards; "Nursing in the dark" emerged after a number of students described the difficulties concerning what they were and were not allowed to say to patients; "Just passing through" emerged as a category through students' description of the constant movement from ward to ward and "Doing the work and being professional" included a discussion of disparate data where students were not always prepared to call the work they were doing 'nursing'. These six categories are all concerned with on-the-job style training, in a hospital environment, within a hierarchical structure, with emphasis upon the role of the student nurse as a pair of hands and not as a supernumerary learner of nursing.

In 1983, Bradby (1989) followed four complete cohorts of female student nurses, in two schools of nursing, during their first year of general training with the aim of identifying any change in the attitudes of students as part of the socialisation process. Bradby uses the term "status passage" to describe the experiences of her subjects in their transition from lay people to first year student nurses. Although the researcher used triangulation of method, the study is restricted in its depth of examination of the issues identified in students' experiences and the length of time during which these experiences occurred.

A comparative study by Wilson and Startup (1991), concerned with the professional socialisation of student nurses, was conducted in three education centres in South Wales during traditional nurse training. The core aim was to discover the roles of teachers and practitioners in establishing the relationship between theory and practice for student nurses and therefore the project draws upon role theory as a theoretical framework. Fundamentally, this research focuses upon the experience of learning nursing skills without consideration of any other contextual data. The term used throughout the report is "socialisation process", which implies that there are recognised stages of development in the process of becoming a nurse. Wilson and Startup adhere to the premiss that there exists a predetermined pattern of events through which students are expected to pass, despite their own evidence which suggests otherwise. Their sample did not undergo an integrated professional socialisation process because they were submitted to conflicting and divergent values between the school of nursing and the wards, an issue which should have been explored more thoroughly because of its potential to influence the development of student nurses. Unfortunately, the emphasis remained upon the expectation of a single predictable process and therefore the data were not fully exploited.

O'Neill, Morrison and McEwen (1993) aimed to compare student socialisation through two different models of nurse education - 'traditional' and 'Project 2000'. Two-hundred and seventy-five students were accessed at various times during the Common Foundation Programme of the Project 2000 course or the first eighteen months of traditional training. The researchers used qualitative methods to compare attitude profiles, perceptions of nursing and experiences in nursing practice. A proportion of students completed each data set consisting of diaries, interviews and questionnaires. Interviews were conducted with a random sample of students from both models of traditional and Project 2000 education. Again qualitative student data were aggregated and a thematic analysis and discussion of the most pertinent issues ensued. There appears to be dependence upon the data to represent the total student population which does not report beyond the Common Foundation Programme. However, the intentions of the study are satisfied in that there is a general evaluation of opinions related to traditional and Project 2000 education by recipients. This complements studies commissioned by the English National Board

(Jowett, Walton and Payne, 1994; Robinson, 1991) which aimed to evaluate the quality of the student experience on Project 2000 courses.

Fifty student nurses were the primary informants in a Canadian study conducted by Day, Field, Campbell and Reutter (1995) during a four year baccalaureate programme. In addition, 81 students completed questionnaires making a total of 131 informants. First, second and third year students were interviewed and re-interviewed in a subsequent year. Content analysis was employed to identify group items and themes using a framework developed by Davis (1975). The student data appear to have been assigned to predetermined themes within this framework; initial innocence, labelled recognition of incongruity, psyching out, role simulation, provisional internalisation and stable internalisation. Whilst this framework is useful for comparing data collected in different studies, in my view, it could prevent the natural emergence of themes. In addition, Davis' theory of "doctrinal conversion" may disregard important current political and social issues relevant to the 1990s. There appears to be a weak rationale for using this framework, resulting in a misfit of theoretical framework to the data generated. However, Day et al. (1995) acknowledge that although students exhibited behaviours are congruent with the stages of Davis' theory of doctrinal conversion, they did not necessarily occur in the sequence that Davis describes. This is an important observation which contributes to the discussion regarding socialisation as a staged process. The idea that students work through a similar process was contested as far back as 1968 by Oleson and Whitaker who claimed that their study revealed that students were active, choice-making individuals who influenced their own socialisation. This supposition is demonstrated throughout written and verbal communications with the participants in my study.

More recently, Macleod Clark, Maben and Jones, (1996) conducted research into perceptions of the philosophy and practice of nursing within the realms of Project 2000. The aims of this research included exploring students', teachers' and practitioners' perceptions in relation to nursing and Project 2000 and identifying the contribution that the Course makes towards the process of professional socialisation. The intention was to generate themes and categories representing 498 students' views which were obtained through questionnaires distributed on three occasions in two case study centres. Macleod Clark et al.'s (1996) study is concerned with professional socialisation and how it is defined and categorised by a large number of students. Using questionnaires, the researchers have determined the direction of questioning, a weakness of previous socialisation studies, in which respondents have been restricted in telling their stories.

8

Gray and Smith (1999) and Philpin (1999) conducted studies during the late 1990s to identify the impact of Project 2000 on the socialisation of Diploma of Higher Education in Nursing Studies students. Philpin, with her interest in aspects of change in the occupational socialisation of nurses, focused upon newly qualified nurses who had undertaken a Project 2000 course and compared their perceptions with those who had been traditionally trained. The intention of this retrospective study was to discover ways that the major change in nurse education had influenced the acquisition of nursing culture. Her findings emphasise the disparity which appears to have existed between nursing education and practice for many years [referred to as the "theory-practice gap" by Bendall, 1974; Holloway and Penson, 1987; Kramer, 1974]. Philpin conducted one set of retrospective interviews [as all participants had been qualified for at least one year and therefore reflected upon their experiences] with her 18 participants. Her main finding was that the nature of the socialisation process related to the work contexts in which it was experienced. In particular, her respondents offered sharply contrasting accounts of their experiences as newly qualified nurses in 'acute' and 'chronic' areas of nursing work. She suggests that her findings "closely parallel" the model of occupational socialisation identified by previous writers such as Melia (1981) and therefore has no reason to contest existing socialisation theory.

Gray and Smith (1999) on the other hand, used a three year longitudinal approach to their investigation which was concerned with exploring the effects of supernumerary status and mentorship on students undertaking clinical practice placements. They used interviews and diaries to elicit the experiences of student nurses on five occasions during their nurse education programme. Gray and Smith developed key categories associated with the professional socialisation of diploma students placing particular emphasis upon effects of supernumerary status and mentorship.

Table 1.1 summarises the characteristics of these socialisation studies for easy comparison.

Comparison of this study with prior studies

From this table it can be seen that several of the early socialisation studies (Bradby, 1983; Melia, 1981; Simpson, 1979; Wyatt, 1978) were only able to sample white females aged between seventeen and twenty-two because this group was representative of recruits to nursing at that time. This has resulted in previous research taking place in contexts

9

Table 1.1   Summary of Socialisation Studies

AUTHOR	DATE	SAMPLE	DATA COLLECTION	PURPOSE/EMPHASIS	ANALYSIS
WYATT	1978	27 young female traditional students.	Interviews in the 2nd or 3rd years of training.	Perceptions of the nurse role. 'Good' and 'bad' features of training.	Descriptive statistics.
SIMPSON	1979	640 white female traditional students.	Questionnaires over a 6 year period.	Measurement of values in nursing.	Aggregation of data for thematic analysis.
MELIA	1981	Various individuals in general nursing branch of traditional training-females aged 17-21yrs.	Interviews at various stages of training.	Ward work; learning and working.	Grounded Theory – Saturation of categories.
BRADBY	1983	4 cohorts of female traditional students.	Observation and interviews after the 1st year of training.	To identify changing attitudes.	Aggregation of data for thematic analysis.
WILSON and STARTUP	1991	43 traditional students, 28 teachers, 35 sisters and charge nurses.	Semi-structured interviews at the beginning of the Course and at the end of the 1st year.	The experience of learning skills.	Aggregation of data for thematic analysis.
O'NEILL, MORRISON and McEWEN	1993	275 Project 2000 and traditional students.	Diaries, interviews and questionnaires at various times, with different students during the CFP.	A comparison of 2 models of nurse education.	Aggregation of data for thematic analysis.
DAY, FIELD, CAMPBELL and REUTTER	1995	50 student informants, 81 additional students.	Interviews with 50 students. Questionnaires for additional 81 students. American baccalaureate programme.	To identify stages of 'doctrinal conversion'.	Predetermined content analysis.
MACLEOD CLARK, MABEN and JONES	1996	498 Project 2000 students accessed at different stages of the Course.	Questionnaires on 3 occasions in 2 case study centres.	To identify the perceptions of the philosophy and practice of nursing.	Aggregation of data for thematic analysis.
PHILPIN	1999	18 newly qualified nurses who had undertaken traditional and Project 2000 courses.	'Retrospective' interviews on 1 occasion.	Aspects of change in the occupational socialisation of nurses.	Grounded Theory – Saturation of categories.
GRAY and SMITH	1999	Project 2000 students.	10 students were interviewed, 7 students kept diaries. Over 3 years on 5 occasions.	To determine the effects of supernumerary status and mentorship on students.	Grounded Theory – Saturation of categories.

where nursing education has been a predominantly female activity involving young women school leavers without previous work experience. This contrasts with the participants in my study who had little in common with each other either in background, age or entry qualifications. Mature students have been actively encouraged to apply for pre-registration diploma courses, tutors believing that students' life experience will enhance their ability to understand the perspective of others in their care. I expected the rightful inclusion of mature and male student nurses in my sample would provide a refreshing insight into their perspective.

Methodologically, many studies have used a grounded theory approach to steer the data collection and analysis strategy. As part of this strategy many of the researchers, except Simpson (1979) and Macleod Clark et al. (1996), have used interviews as the main data collection method which, in my view, means that the researchers have satisfied their own agenda and not that of the participants. This contrasts with my adoption of hermeneutically compatible techniques which gave participants control over what they chose to tell me about their lifeworld in order to illustrate their development over a three year period. Students were empowered to convey the meaning of their experiences to me, directing and determining how the next data collection phase would be conducted. Thus, a more flexible and responsive approach was adopted.

The continuity of data collection phases with each participant and the use of multiple methods, which enabled students to tell their stories, has produced a richer and contextually more meaningful narrative. This constitutes an original approach within nurse socialisation literature.

I would contend that the use of multiple methods enhances the truth value of qualitative data; Melia's (1981) restricted use of interviews as a method has resulted in the collection and presentation of a variety of student experiences in isolation without identifying connections between individuals' experiences.

None of the other researchers represented in Table 1.1 make links between individual sets of data. The majority analyse the data as an aggregate in order to determine themes, without identifying the personal traits, needs, experiences or social background of students, which may affect the way in which they develop during their nurse education programme. Although many topics have been raised and discussed in these studies, the meaning that experiences have for individuals has been largely ignored. The focus of my study lies within the individual orientations, experience and relatedness of the Self to the occupation; education and practice are contexts within which these developments

11

occur.

The majority of studies noted above utilise or depend upon the socialisation model which values the 'professional product' as dictated by society. My intention is not to claim representation of the student population through the volunteer sample in my study, but to illuminate examples of ways in which the professional role of the nurse may be undertaken. Having been involved in the process of my participants' development, I would dispute claims that socialisation occurs as a linear process, whereby all socialisees pass through identified, recognised stages of 'becoming'.

Finally, although there are apparent similarities between some of the studies summarised above (Gray and Smith, 1999; O'Neill, Morrison and McEwen, 1993) and my own, all being concerned with student nurse development and utilising data collected on several occasions, the purpose of these studies differ significantly from mine. However, all the studies mentioned within this brief section have informed and reminded me that nursing work is not homogenous and there is room for all contributions within the socialisation or occupational 'becoming' literature.

After exposure to this literature and much more related to nurse education; selection and recruitment; attrition and wastage; the role of the teacher, mentor, supervisor, preceptor; Project 2000 reforms, documents and evaluations, the aims for my study became apparent;

- To illuminate experiences of student nurses undertaking the Diploma of Higher Education in Nursing Studies course in an attempt to understand the meaning they assign to those experiences.
- To portray the learning milieu in which students 'become' nurses through a hermeneutic analysis of their descriptions and stories.

Having situated my research amongst other socialisation literature and identified the aims for my study, it is appropriate to discuss the structure and style of this book.

About this book - style and form; a guide for the reader

I have taken heed of Laurel Richardson (1992, 1994) who advises qualitative researchers to write from the Self so that individual voices, including that of the researcher, may be identified within the text. She reminds us that, unlike quantitative work, which can carry its meaning in tables and summaries, qualitative work depends upon people's reading of it. Qualitative research has to be read, not scanned; its meaning is in the reading. I endeavoured to keep this in mind whilst writing the original thesis.

Woods (1999) also stresses that writing in qualitative research is particularly important because its value rests on description, narrative, argument and persuasion, unlike quantitative research with its reliance on statistical and technical instruments.

Writing, as Evans (1997) asserts, occupies a great deal of time during the process of conducting research. She identifies the different purposes and forms which writing occupies during the course of study for a PhD; field notes, initial writing up of the research process, tentative drafts of chapters, transcriptions, publications and conference papers. Each of these writing activities requires a certain, expected style of presentation in order for the writing to be effective, accepted and believed.

Closs (1994) states that;

> The English should be as simple and concise as it can be without losing any intricacies of meaning. Jargon which adds nothing to an explanation should be avoided, although technical terminology which is essential to give precise explanation may be needed.
>
> (Closs, 1994, p44)

Whilst I have searched for the simplest, most direct way to express my thoughts in this thesis, reference is necessary to the work of Heidegger (1962) which, in itself, is very complex. Whenever I have used Heidegger's terminology, or referred to his concepts, my understanding and interpretation have been explained to enable the reader to begin from a similar point of reference. I have been comforted by Spiegelberg (1969), who claims that no reader without an exceptional command of German can expect to fathom the sense and full connotations of Heidegger's language. I have found it particularly difficult to grasp the meaning and intention of Heidegger's terms, but Dilworth (1989) believes there is nothing sacred in any of the past philosophical systems that renders them impervious to reinterpretation. He does however, maintain that it would be foolish to think that anyone could refute or deconstruct any of the great philosophical texts and it is not my intention to do so in this book. It could be that the delay in English translations of Heidegger's work is related to the primary difficulty of interpretation; indeed Spiegelberg refers to native Germans being "stymied" by Heidegger's way of writing;

For Heidegger has a way of not only forming new terms based on absolute root meanings, but of using existing words for new and unheard of purposes without providing a glossary as a key or introducing his new uses by explicit definitions.

(Spiegelberg, 1982, p273)

I have also chosen not to provide reference dates for Heidegger (1962) and Kelly (1955) each time I use their work or a direct quotation, because I have done so frequently. Where I have used their work, I refer to the page number. Whilst the original sources for these seminal works are 1962 and 1955 respectively, I have used the modern versions of the texts which are reprinted, but not rewritten. The page numbers relate to the modern versions for Heidegger (1997) and Kelly (1991).

All other references are arranged, if necessary, in alphabetical order and not in date order.

Whenever I refer to the Project 2000 course as 'the Course', I have used a capital 'C' to distinguish it from other uses of the word 'course'.

Using the "I" word

Charmaz and Mitchell (1997) talk of the 'myth of silent authorship' which refers to qualitative studies in the past being written by a disembodied voice. It appeared that all human dynamism (p193) between researcher and participants during the course of data collection was lost in the written account. Woods (1999) claims that it is now customary for qualitative researchers to include some biographical details in recognition of their personal histories having some bearing on the research outcome and product and I have introduced myself through simple verse at the beginning of Chapter 5.

Webb (1992) believes that nursing, as a relatively young academic discipline, has attempted to establish respect and credibility by imitating longer-established disciplines which have encouraged the use of writing in the third person. The novice writer and even those with more experience, painfully construct their essays using excruciatingly tortuous sentences to portray what 'the writer', 'the author' or 'the student' think. I agree with Webb that this style of writing is appropriate when referring to a generally accepted body of knowledge and when reviewing a subject in the light of available evidence.

But using 'it is thought' rather than 'I think' and 'data were collected' instead of 'I collected data' conveys an impression that the ideas being discussed are neutral and value-free. This of course, cannot be the case in a study which uses Self as the major instrument in the research. All forms of research involve a certain amount of social interaction but, with interpretive approaches, researchers invest and divulge much of 'themselves' in their research. Using "I" throughout this book may be provocative to some in relation to questions of rigour. In order to address these challenges, I have plotted my decision trail in the methodology chapter to enable the reader to trace my thought processes and reasons for choosing various methods and techniques.

Another reason why third person writing is inappropriate in interpretive enquiry, is 'reflexivity' which requires the researcher to reflect continuously throughout the research process on their actions, participants' reactions to them and how they are collecting, analysing and interpreting data. It is essential for reflections to be offered as part of the research, otherwise it might not be possible to evaluate it thoroughly.

Finally, within this study, trying to put descriptions of the processes and my involvement in them into the traditional third person writing would not only be awkward but untrue to the philosophical premiss of hermeneutic phenomenology which informs the study.

A decision about footnotes

Woods (1999) comments on the use of 'footnotes' which contain information that is thought to be relevant, but would get in the way of a developing narrative or argument if placed in the body of the text. I have chosen not to use footnotes in this book as they can be distracting and it is my belief that if a footnote is indicated, the essential information should be worked into the text or, as an alternative, placed in the appendices.

Identifying 'voices' in the text

The production of this text has of course, been influenced by the voices of the actors within the research. It would be confusing and inappropriate to give each of them a type font of their own. For clarity, when quoting them I have used *Italics* to identify the voices of practitioners, tutors and students in this text. My reflections, taken from my dictaphone and my own dialogue, appear in type font 'Arial'. I hope that this explanation will help the reader discern the voices.

Evans (1997) cites Packwood and Sikes (1996) who warn of the situation in which experimentation and "stylistic attempts to represent voice" (p338) can become of greater importance than the reality of the text. I agree with Evans that the issue is not the desire to experiment with the text, more it is a personal need to represent the voices of participants in the study and my own lived experience of the research process.

Using poetry

As an introduction and conclusion to Part IV, I have used poetry as a means of capturing the essence of students' perceptions of themselves at the beginning and end of the Diploma of Higher Education in Nursing Studies course. Richardson (1994) argues the merits of poetry and comments on nine short poems she has written which inspired me to use the words of my participants and construct verses to represent their situation and perceptions. Richardson argues that this method, involving a series of poems, is far more successful than more traditional methods of conveying the sense of 'lived experience' to the reader. However, Bailey (1996, p108) notes that this form of writing is not for everyone and that some readers may prefer a standard style of introduction. For me, the use of poetry is a more poignant way of capturing the character of the students and is also a more economical and interesting use of words. Richardson's case for using poetry convinced me that it was an appropriate way to represent the students and, although I may not be poetically gifted, I am content with the outcome. Poetry also 'fits' with the philosophical approach used to guide this study which recommends alternative ways of viewing lifeworld (Richardson, 1992).

Parts and chapters

The content of this book is arranged in chapters within parts. Part I, which comprises this current chapter, is concerned with introducing the reader to the text and the subject area for investigation.

Within Part II, Chapters 2 and 3 convey the philosophical underpinnings and methodological processes and considerations so that the reader might gain insight into the reasons why I used particular methods and techniques for gathering and analysing data.

Part III is concerned with contextualising and portraying the panorama of the study. Within it, Chapter 4 summarises interviews with practitioners and focus groups with nurse tutors, in order to develop the context of the study against which the students' perspectives are presented later. In Chapter 5, I expose my Self as a multidimensional Being - comprising a Practitioner, Educationalist and Researcher presence. As these Selves are responsible for the planning, development, and subsequent analysis within this study, I felt that it was important to allow them a separate chapter.

Chapters 6 to 10, within Part IV, unfold the phenomena of 'Becoming a Nurse'. These chapters utilise hermeneutic phenomenological concepts as their titles - these are explained in each chapter.

Finally, within Part V, Chapter 11 summarises and concludes the study and I take the opportunity to reflect upon the process as a whole. I consider the implications of this study for nurse education, practice and research and suggest possible lines for future enquiry. I also bring the text to a close by summarising the original contribution it makes to nurse education and practice and suggest potential publications which can be generated from it.

Summary

In this chapter, I have endeavoured to lay the foundation for the study and give the reader a flavour of the literature which informed and motivated me to pursue this line of enquiry.

It is evident from the material presented here, that previous socialisation studies have been driven by traditional views concerning socialisation - that is, socialisees undergo a similar staged process to one another, regardless of age, gender and background. In these studies data were subjected to aggregation and analysis to saturate categories and produce common themes. I am unaware of any other studies within nurse socialisation literature which use a hermeneutic analysis as an alternative approach.

I have also given the reader some practical direction through this text in the hope that their journey through the work is logical and progressive.

In the next part, I intend to explicate how hermeneutic phenomenology has provided direction for me, and also how the research was planned and conducted.

Part II

Philosophical and Methodological Foundations

In Part I, I provided an overview of the relevant literature concerned with the socialisation of student nurses into the professional role. It was evident that although the literature explored important aspects of becoming a nurse, individuals' journeys and experiences had not been explicated because data had been collectively analysed and researchers rarely followed a group of students consistently through their education programme.

> There is a temptation to view socialisation as consisting of discrete slices of time, one after the other. To do so is risky, for the observer may think a series of delimited time-bound events add up to the whole process. Such a procedure may unwittingly over-emphasise selected events and reactions to them or it may fail to identify the most significant times when processes are begun or stabilised.
>
> (Simpson, 1979, p16)

Much of the available socialisation material has been based upon studies conducted using young, white females in the research sample which has provided a somewhat narrow representation of the applicants to current nurse education courses.

The intention of Part II is to demonstrate how I chose to use Heideggerian Hermeneutic Phenomenology in conjunction with Kelly's Personal Construct Theory in order to gain an understanding of what it was like to be a student nurse on a Project 2000 course. The emphasis in this part is upon the underpinning philosophies and the processes employed which gave me direction and the research process its structure. In Chapter 2, I pay particular attention to how my thought processes evolved using hermeneutics and how I relied upon my background as a nurse to make links between 'care' as a physical and emotional act and 'care' as a philosophical existential.

It is important to note that I do not claim that this work is either a sociological or psychological analysis. Hermeneutics is described in the next chapter as an approach which focuses upon understanding the meaning of experience to participants. To satisfy this requirement I have drawn on both sociology and psychology to make sense of students' experiences within a hermeneutic phenomenological framework.

In Chapter 3, I take the reader along the decision trail of the methodology and describe the processes involved in collecting and analysing data whilst adhering to the demands of a hermeneutic approach.

2 Informing Philosophies

In this chapter, I intend to set out the philosophical foundations of the study so that the reader might gain insight into the guiding perspectives, beliefs and values that I have endeavoured to satisfy and maintain throughout the research process.

It is necessary, in this chapter, to illuminate the overarching influence that ontology has had upon this study and then to explain how hermeneutics as an interpretive approach has permitted me to develop a thorough and appropriate strategy. I shall justify the choice of Martin Heidegger, in particular his writings from *Being and Time* (1962), which advocate a hermeneutic phenomenological approach to investigating the everydayness of being and becoming. Links will be made between his philosophical stance and those of nurse theorists, such as Leininger (1988), Parse (1981), Peplau (1952) and Watson (1979) who have used phenomenology to inform their models for nursing practice. These models may be more familiar and understandable to the reader with a nursing background than Heidegger's work and may be helpful in building a more comprehensive rationale.

Finally, I shall endeavour to make clear the connection between personal construct theory and phenomenology and how I have integrated them to provide a strong philosophical structure for this research.

The overarching ontological influence

The motivation for this study stemmed from a desire to gain understanding of the meaning of what it was like to be a student on a Project 2000, Diploma of Higher Education in Nursing Studies course. In order to satisfy this intent, firstly I needed to discover a philosophy congruent with my own perspective, historicality [background] and horizon [frame of reference] and secondly, I needed a philosophical framework to provide direction and focus during the research process. To find a 'method' to satisfy these two requirements seemed to be the starting point.

Heidegger (1982, pp320-330) explains what constitutes ontology and discusses the difference between 'Being' as an 'existential' [experiences through existence – philosophy] and 'being' as in 'human beings' [which describes the physiological existence, through positive science].

Ontology is about understanding the state of 'Being' and what it is like 'to be' in any given situation. Heidegger (pp28-35) describes the ability and potential 'to be' as 'Dasein'. The basic meaning of 'Dasein' is 'Being there', the requirement of which is to be conscious of one's existence. A special distinction of Dasein is that it has an understanding of itself in its Being, a sense of reality and a participation in the creation of personal and social knowledge (Guba, 1990). Koch (1996) reports that the Dasein concept of a person's 'Being-in-the-world' necessitates a view that the person and the world are co-constituted, this being an indissoluble unity. As such, an individual makes sense of the world from within their own existence and not while detached from it. These beliefs form the basis of ontology. Reason and Rowan (1981) claim;

> We have to learn to think dialectically, to view reality as a process, always emerging through a self-contradictory development, always becoming; knowing this reality is neither subjective nor objective, it is both wholly independent of me and wholly dependent on me.
>
> (Reason and Rowan, 1981, p241)

This is an especially apt and interesting tenet from which to operate when the intent is to gain insight into others' development during a process of becoming.

Ontology contrasts to epistemology, a concern for the nature and theory of knowledge and how it is acquired. Rather than searching for a foundation of knowledge as in epistemology, ontology is driven by the need to understand structures of reality as people experience it. This was a most attractive proposition and one which I believed would provide me with a platform to capture the essence of being a student nurse.

Other nurse researchers have identified differences between the ontological and epistemological aspects of care such as in research on hope for those with disease (Kylma and Vehvilainen-Julkunen, 1997). This enabled researchers to describe the affective, temporal and relational dimensions of hope in addition to the essence and distinctive characteristics of hope. Similarly, Holden (1991, (1)) analyses the attributions, contributions and resolutions of caring and discusses the ontological anxiety experienced by nurses in association with suffering and loss (p895). Knowledge gained through this type of ontological enquiry is particularly relevant to nursing practice as it identifies affective and aesthetic aspects of care which may not be exposed in research which uses a more traditional approach.

Heidegger explains that Dasein's ontological constitution is rooted in time and temporality (1982, p229), which suggests that we have an interpretation of the connectedness between what has been, what is, and what might be. Again, this perspective is appropriate when trying to identify personal and professional development in individuals and when seeking to obtain an overview of the meaning of that development.

Nolan, Brown and Crawford (1998) examined the implications of Nietzsche's ideas for the caring professions, in particular those involved in caring for people with mental health problems. They claim that using ontology to understand mental ill-health provides carers with a perspective on changing individuals.

> In Nietzsche's view there is an uneasy relationship between ourselves and our history. We can come to terms with it by accepting it and transcending it. This is achieved by constructing who we are in the future. Happiness can only exist when we forget the past. Too much preoccupation with the past induces pessimism and this can stifle and thwart our progress ... The past is what we were, the present is what we are, but who we are is in the future.
>
> (Nolan, Brown and Crawford, 1998, p254)

In this study I have utilised phenomenology [the name for the method of ontology], in an attempt to understand the lifeworld of student nurses and the meaning they assign to their experiences during the Diploma of Higher Education in Nursing Studies course.

Why hermeneutic phenomenology?

As a contemporary philosophy and research methodology, hermeneutics is concerned with the thick description which emanates from people's detailed stories of their experiences in their everyday understanding of Being-in-the-world. Hermeneutics is described as a method which facilitates interpretation of texts within context (Honderich, 1995, p352), where 'texts' refers to sources of information in addition to the written word. Elliston and McCormick (1977) claim that even 'imagining' is a basic hermeneutic technique. This enables textual interpretation and, according to Dilthey (1976), provides access to meaning not only of written texts, but of signs and symbols of all sorts, social practices, historical action, works of art and future expectations.

It is van Manen's (1990, p9) belief that hermeneutics aims to interpret experiences within a given context without classifying or abstracting them; this contrasts to 'pure' phenomenology which seeks to describe meaning. For this reason, hermeneutics has become attractive to nurse researchers as a research approach, but Leonard (1989) states that too often researchers quickly seize on the method without considering the more profoundly important philosophical assumptions that undergird the method, or whether those assumptions are consistent with the researcher's own view of what it means to be a human being. Blumer (1969, p25) concurs with this opinion and adds;

> The relationship between the research act and the theoretical framework is critical. This picture sets the selection and formulation of problems, the determination of what are data, the means to be used in getting data, the kinds of relations sought between data and the forms in which propositions are cast.
>
> (Blumer, 1969, p25)

Indeed, Koch (1995) criticises the research of Benner and Wrubel (1989), [which set a precedent in nurse education for assessing students' development in clinical practice], because the participant/subject/patient is always 'situated' but the researcher remains aloof. She further notes that these authors do not discuss the application of the hermeneutic circle to their work, thus excluding what is one of the central notions of Heidegger's existential hermeneutics. The hermeneutic circle is a metaphor used to describe the dynamic movement which occurs between parts and the whole of the text whilst seeking 'verstehen' [understanding]. The researcher constantly weaves in and out of data sets whilst conducting the research reflexively, so that the researcher's Self is central to understanding and interpretation. Indeed, being explicit about the way the researcher accesses the circle is part of the validation process in a hermeneutic study. Heidegger gave the circle an ontological connection to his notion of Dasein and fore-understanding (Bleicher, 1980 p267). Koch (1995) sees disregard for the central notion of researcher and subject being situated in the world as "hermeneutics practised outside the circle" (p834).

I believe that my background greatly influenced the analysis and therefore should be included in the data. Dreyfus (1987) writes "from the beginning the person is amongst it all, being in it, coping with it" (p254). Inclusion of my background and experience associated with nursing and nurse education has, to some extent, protected against the imposition of arbitrary assumptions and pre-suppositions. By making my fore-understandings conscious and by examining their origin, I believe that I have engaged in an insightful process of metatheoretical reflection which is considered to be a form of enquiry itself (Morrow, 1994). Although a hermeneutic approach actively encourages researchers to expose their perspective, there is a contrasting belief that prior knowledge of a situation, preconceived ideas and personal bias may be imposed upon data (Beck, 1991, p19; Rose, 1990, p59). Crotty (1996, p19) cites several nurse researchers who believe that 'bracketing', [that is the 'putting aside' of these fore-understandings and suspending beliefs; also referred to in other texts as 'epoche' (Husserl, 1970), 'presuppositionlessness' (Crotty, 1996) or 'phenomenological reduction' (Moustakas, 1994)], makes the researcher free to be receptive to the participants and keeps their meaning separate from that of the researcher. In this way, they argue, the data are accepted uncritically as given. But, if it is genuinely the case that phenomenological research is the study of the lived experience and phenomenology's purpose is to seek a fuller understanding through description, reflection and self awareness (Ray, 1990), then producing a phenomenological narrative that reflects this fuller understanding of the lived experience is essential. However, there is evidence to suggest that nurse researchers find it very difficult to make a decision whether to bracket or not (Jasper, 1994; Rose, Beeby and Parker, 1995; Taylor, 1993; Walters, 1995). Lipson (1997) views this as a paradoxical struggle for the researcher, "to both keep yourself in there and out at the same time" (p23). It is acknowledged that during data collection phases, interactions between the researcher and researched occur which often lead to other relationships being formed outside the research (Bergum, 1991).

Bleicher (1980) criticises the notion of bracketing because, he claims, the circle cannot be avoided, rather it is a matter of getting into it properly as it contains the possibility of original insight; understanding is not the result of a correct procedure; rather it is found in the hermeneutic circle. Beck (1994) believes that the values of the researcher, rather than obscuring the data from respondents, make the research meaningful to the consumer, particularly as in my research where I expect that consumers will almost certainly be those with concern for nursing and nurse education or with similar, related interest and frame of reference.

According to Gadamer (1975, pp271-274), understanding for the researcher occurs through a fusion of horizons which is reasoning between pre-understanding of the situation, the interpretive framework and the sources of information. The implication for hermeneutic enquiry is that research participants are also giving their self-interpreted

25

construction of their situation. The result could be many constructions or multiple realities, including the researcher's construction of the same phenomena. This occurs because we all have a conscious engagement in the world. If this is so, complete reduction leading to bracketing, as Merleau-Ponty (1964) points out, is not possible. From Gadamer's perspective, it is actually an advantage not to be freed from prejudice in a hermeneutic situation, as being first and foremost an everyday actor, gives the ability to understand that which is different (Deertz, 1978).

Beech (1999) discusses the origins of bracketing and describes the activity as "the abeyance of all preconceptions on behalf of the researcher" (p36). He argues that it is an important methodological principle which should be adhered to if one is to gain authentic insights into the lifeworld of another. However, there seem to be some misunderstandings and indeed, some misinterpretations of the term bracketing in and around the nursing research literature by authors who claim to have bracketed. This is not surprising if, as Beech suggests (p39), there is more than one way to bracket. He tries to describe the processes involved in bracketing which appear complex and, at times, confused and unintelligible.

Why Heideggerian hermeneutic phenomenology?

Husserl (1962) is generally acknowledged as the founder of phenomenology and was the first to suggest bracketing as a means whereby researchers should look at things as they actually appear; without influence from preconceptions, biases or judgements. Heidegger has contrasting values, in that he believes the researcher contributes, through experience, values and presuppositions about the phenomena being explored. Both the phenomenological philosophies of Husserl [transcendental phenomenology] and Heidegger [hermeneutic phenomenology] were considered as a basis for my research, but it is evident that they provide different philosophical underpinnings for researchers' methodologies and thus have different implications for research. Husserlian phenomenology conceptualises the individual as a subject in a world of objects and is primarily concerned with epistemological issues, whereas Heideggerian philosophy focuses upon the ontological issues related to what it means to be a person. In Heidegger's work, the hermeneutic account of 'verstehen' no longer refers to the question of how the subjective world is constituted in consciousness, as it does for Husserl; the focus is on the question of what Being is, or rather how human life is itself a process and product of

26

theories of interpretation. In *Being and Time*, Heidegger's early work, the question is not how Being can be understood, but how understanding is Being (Gadamer, 1977, p49).

There are many interpretations and critiques of Heidegger's work (Dreyfus, 1991; Guignon, 1996; Kockelmans, 1986; Mulhall, 1990) which decipher the language, translate and interpret his meanings in relation to Being. It is my interpretation that it is not Heidegger's goal to explore meanings of everyday practices in a simplistic way; grouping, categorising and describing those everyday practices. Instead, as Crotty (1996, p81) notes, Heidegger wishes to explore the meaning of those everyday practices to the individual.

Like Heidegger, Gadamer (1975) has no place in his philosophical framework for techniques of bracketing; they also share a belief about the central notions of hermeneutics. Gadamer rejected the notion of eliminating one's own prejudices and developed the concept of the 'fusion of horizons'. Gadamer explains the metaphor of an horizon as "the wide superior vision that the person who is seeking to understand must have". He believes that prejudices contribute to a person's horizon and this is being continuously formed through reflection and a consciousness of one's 'historicity'; that is, interpretation occurs against a backdrop of the researcher's ontological relation to their own history (Koch, 1995). I refer to 'horizon' in later chapters where I make an attempt to draw contrasts and similarities between my own horizon or frame of reference, and those of others who have a part in this research. I have found the notion of horizon and how it can be extended or stunted especially useful in explaining movement and development of particular understandings and beliefs over time I like the image of my own horizon changing as a result of being enlightened and I hope to have captured some evidence of this in Chapter 5 where I disclose my emerging Selves whilst conducting this study.

Rejected philosophical options

On an epistemological level, critical theory, like hermeneutics, has attempted to show the limits of the objectifying methods of natural science. One of Habermas' (1987) goals has been to install critical theory in order to promote emancipation. The concern for class structure and social conditions for health and health care reform, issues of multiculturalism and cultural sensitivity, and the struggle against oppression have seen critical theory grow as a preferred methodology within nursing research literature. Such facilitation of emancipation by the researcher did not appeal to me because of the risk of adopting a paternalistic role with the student participants. One of my aims in this study has been to try to maintain an equable power balance; often it has been out of my control as students are aware of the power tensions in clinical practice settings where they are subordinate as a result of being a transient workforce. Although critical theory was an option as a philosophical foundation to this study, I was aware that taking on the required facilitative, almost therapeutic role could have resulted in conflict at any stage during the study. Habermas (1971, p310) stresses that critical theory proves its validity only by addressing itself to victims of domination and eliciting self-reflection in which the victim recognises themself in the theory. Critical theory places an emphasis on illuminating and relieving oppression and encompasses Habermas' communication and political action through education; a process which also moves in a circle.

Choosing to reject critical theory as a methodology for this study does not mean that I have denied the conflicts which exist along the seams of lifeworld. Rather, using hermeneutics, I have sought to gain understanding of these conflicts throughout the process of becoming a nurse, from the student's perspective. I take from Habermas the importance of the emancipatory project and share the hope that hermeneutics might develop characteristics of an emancipatory discipline in the future (Nicholson cited by Silverman, 1991, p161). To integrate hermeneutics and critical theory it would be necessary to attend to the remit and role of the researcher in order to preserve the integrity of the hermeneutic circle [see Mendelson, 1979 for a thorough contrast of hermeneutics and critical theory].

Foucault's theory of interpretation (Visker, 1991), aims to reveal connections between power relations and knowledge. Through a basic understanding of his work, I have identified a discrepancy between hermeneutics and Foucault's theory, despite important similarities. Whilst Heidegger claims an allegiance to the hermeneutic circle to facilitate understanding of the meaning of phenomena to the individual and between individuals [thus it is self-validating], Foucault advocates understanding discourse produced through institutions and practices, rather than means for exploring individuals' experience. Stern (1985) implies that Heidegger's hermeneutics is 'oceanic' [all encompassing] as opposed to 'restricted' [limited] (p290) as in Foucault's interpretive stance. He writes;

Such theories are either circular or self-defeating. The charge of circularity is raised in connection with the problem of the hermeneutic circle: understanding a symbol depends on understanding a larger unit, which in turn requires understanding its constituent symbols. Each interpretation creates the facts it wants to explain; we can no longer speak about conflicting interpretations of the same text; finally, we can no longer distinguish between interpretations and what they are interpretations of.

(Stern, 1985, p290)

My understanding is that Foucault believes interpretation need not be context bound, unlike Heidegger who advocates a strong association between phenomena and the contexts in which they occur. He believes that by so doing, meaning is made more relevant, applicable and associated but Foucault implies that this produces an unstable interpretation because meaning and interpretation are not distinguished. I would argue that, providing the phenomena are described and interpreted and the researcher's horizon is declared, the audience is able to understand the text, in context, through their own horizon. In other words, they can make decisions about all aspects of the research if they have sufficient information about the decision trail made by the researcher. This is addressed in the following chapter on methodology.

Another choice of ontological framework which might have suited the needs of this study is Sartre's (1996) 'philosophy of human freedom' which proposes that one could never understand what it is like to be a human being if one does not understand the extent of human freedom. Being free, for Sartre, is the ultimate 'existential' and one which expounds the nature of human life. In his arguments within 'Being and Nothingness' (1969, 1978, 1996) Sartre demonstrates a commitment to a 'psycho-analysis of things'. This is probably where Sartre's and my intentions depart. My intentions for this study include a hermeneutic analysis of the data collected in order to provide an interpretation of the meaning student nurses assign to various experiences in nursing practice and education within a framework of ontology rather than psychology. Sartre's emphasis is also on the moral aspects of Being, a perspective I did not want to address in this study. Stewart (1995, p314) also believes that Sartre's theory lends itself to criticism because he seems to have confined freedom to mere freedom of thought and by so doing has made it such that we are always free. This contrasts to the view of Merleau-Ponty (1948) who claims that freedom can only make sense if it is accompanied and empowered by real possibility: "no effective freedom exists without some power" (p148). Indeed, Heidegger states that Dasein is never free from 'Being - in' (p84) because it always encounters the world and has no choice about it. This implication of Heidegger's that we are all in constant

29

interaction with the environment and with each other was more attractive as a premiss than Sartre's claim to total conscious freedom.

I also feel the need to state at this juncture that it is my intention to utilise Heidegger's philosophical works, mainly from *Being and Time* as a foundation for this study and not to refer to the possible political consequences of his philosophy as outlined by Holmes (1996). This association of Heidegger [like Nietzsche], with the Nazi party has lent his work morally suspect connotations. Claims about Heidegger's commitment to Nazism and the controversy associated with his apparent anti-humanism are debated elsewhere in the literature (Cushing, 1994; Thompson, 1994).

'Care' as central to Heideggerian and nursing philosophies

Various ideologies of care have been identified (James, 1992) and caring is thought to be the essence and unifying domain of nursing (Leininger, 1988; Watson, 1988). It is not surprising therefore that as a nurse and nurse educator, I have been attracted by Heidegger's focus on care. Within the realms of Heidegger's hermeneutic phenomenology, caring and care feature as fundamental elements and are seen to constitute the whole Being of Dasein.

Being-in-the-world-with-others, experiencing anxiety, recognising potential, all mean that essentially we care. Heidegger (pp235-244) explains that Dasein is always absorbed in the world because of its concern with others and itself, and gives the example of care being manifested as "political action" or "taking a rest and enjoying oneself". If one is willing to do something, care shows through. Using the expression of care [sorge] as a basic ontological phenomenon, Heidegger develops his theory of interpretation around care in much the same way as Sartre uses freedom as the central tenet of his theory of interpretation.

Recognition should be given to the fact that nursing does not have a monopoly on caring. Sourial (1997) identifies the differences between personal and professional properties of caring and attempts to discover all the uses of the concept of caring in the nursing literature. These include the ethics of caring; instrumental and affective ways of caring; caring traits; perceptions of caring; organisational and quality effects of caring.

I am not the first nurse to be drawn to Heideggerian hermeneutics through the concept of caring. In her study, Taylor (1994, pp181-200) utilises Heidegger's expression of care as Being and also the work of

30

Campbell (1984) suggests that human caring, as the essence of nursing, is expressed as a form of moderated love. The basic premiss of Taylor's study is that human caring is a perceived state of Being through which people express their connectedness to one another in everyday ways befitting their relationships. Taylor concludes that caring manifests as therapeutic interpersonal relationships which make the phenomenon of illness manageable for people who need nursing care. Interestingly she suggests that nurses may be tempted to hide in their professional roles, thereby diminishing the value of their essential ordinariness as humans in the nursing encounter - the very point that Heidegger emphasises as being important in his philosophy - care as the core of Being and not just a professional role. Indeed, Nelms (1996) believes that often the meaning of caring presence in nursing and human caring in general is so deeply embedded in our consciousness and cultural practices that its presence is invisible or taken for granted. Also using a Heideggerian hermeneutic approach to her research, Nelms set out to illuminate nurses' shared practices and common meanings of living a caring presence in nursing. The match between choice of philosophical approach and the intent of the study in Nelms' paper serves as an excellent example of how important fittingness and congruency are, and I consider her research contributes to an understanding of the meaning of Being in general terms as well as having specific application to nursing.

Parallels between Heideggerian and nursing philosophies

In Chapter 8 in this thesis, 'Being-in-the-world-with-others' is explored in relation to students' caring presence with patients, clients and relatives. Like Nelms, I have attempted to capture the essence of caring and how the students embraced themselves as caring beings; they also embraced others as beings in need of care and, by so doing, revealed the essence of nursing. Other nurse researchers, with an interest in care as the root of nursing, include Johns (1996), Macleod (1994), Maltby, Drury and Fischer-Rasmussen (1995), Roach (1992), Street (1992) and Taylor (1994).

Parse's (1992) concept of 'true presence' and Benner and Wrubel's (1989) construction of stress and coping in health and illness, use hermeneutic phenomenology to portray nursing activities which matter and manifest as caring presence.

The ability to presence oneself, to be with a patient in a way that acknowledges your shared humanity, is the basis of nursing as a caring presence.

(Benner and Wrubel, 1989, p13)

Parse demonstrates her allegiance to hermeneutics through her cogent argument that intersubjective participation is the only valid and legitimate means by which human becoming can be understood (Parse, 1993, p41). Parse's theory is based upon a set of assumptions which encompass the central belief that events and people mutually shape and influence one another. Parse talks of "synchronising rhythms" (p41) which refers to the ebb and flow of human encounters and the struggle and triumph of everyday living with others. Within her nursing model there is also a dimension of 'mobilising transcendence' (Parse, 1990) which refers to ever-changing situations in life. She believes that it is the nurse's task to help patients and families to prepare for changing health patterns and plan to reach 'possible' Selves. It is also Parse's intention to structure meaning multidimensionally so that understanding is enabled through an illumination of perceptions, gestures, expressions and language and this contributes to the development of her theory of human becoming. This type of intent is typical of a hermeneutic approach to seeking meaning.

Like Parse, Watson (1979) believes that intersubjectivity between researcher and researched, observer and observed, and nurse and patient, must occur - she contends that the act of care must, necessarily, involve transcendental togetherness between the patient-person and the nurse-person characterised by co-operation and connectedness (Watson, 1985, pp58-59) and this forms the basis of her theory of transpersonal care.

Parse and Watson share the vision that human life, or being-in-the-world, is the appropriate subject matter for nursing. In addition, detachment and objectivity are not only incongruent with the subject matter of nursing, as Parse points out, but they constitute the very antithesis of Watson's caring ideal. Whilst Watson focuses on the existential phenomenological and spiritual basis of caring and sees caring as the ethical and moral ideal of nursing, Leininger's (1988) theoretical/conceptual model reflects an anthropological approach to viewing individuals within a cultural context where caring patterns differ transculturally. She classifies a number of constructs into a taxonomy of human caring, developed to assist nurses conceptualise, order and study types of caring phenomena. Both Watson's 'transpersonal caring' and Leininger's 'transcultural caring' contribute to nursing knowledge by exploring universal aspects of human care as well as specific care particular to an individual, family, institution, society or culture.

Heidegger argues that having concern or care as part of Being involves a multiplicity of activities such as the following;

having to do with something, producing something, attending to something and looking after it, making use of something, giving something up and letting it go, undertaking, accomplishing, evincing, interrogating, considering, discussing, determining ...

(Heidegger, p83)

These activities are fundamental to the role of the nurse through their committed involvement in patients' and clients' existential life situations and these present a challenge to 'do something about it', in order to make certain difficult decisions about care.

Peplau (1952, 1988, 1994, 1996) also became acquainted with phenomenological ideas through the work of humanistic psychologists and drew on the ideas of Maslow (1954), May (1969) and Rogers (1942). Peplau believes that the only way to discover the authentic meaning of nursing's task is to examine particular care relationships and interactions, rooted in time and place (Peplau, 1994). Through these relationships and interactions, nurses attend to the 'somethings' stated above by Heidegger. Peplau's 'interpersonal relations' model acknowledges that the experience of proximity and distance, unity and separation, equality and difference - the rejection of any aspiration to complete transparency - means that nurses respect their patients as having unique value in themselves (Gastmans, 1998, p1317), a central tenet of Heidegger's hermeneutics.

Consideration, congruency and integration of Kelly's and Heidegger's philosophies

My first acquaintance with Kelly's Personal Construct Theory (1955) was during my search for appropriate methods and techniques which, when used, would satisfy a hermeneutic requirement and the aims of the study. Kelly's theory of personality started with a combination of two simple notions; first, that people might be better understood if they were viewed in the perspective of enduring time rather than in a flicker of passing moments; and second, that people contemplate in their own personal way the stream of events which occur during a lifetime. Within this interplay of notions, it may then be possible to discover ways in which people restructure their lives as a result of experience.

Kelly refers to the patterns which people assign to understandings about their lives as 'constructs'. 'Construing' the world means that people are enabled to chart a course of behaviour in response to, and as a result of, previous similar experiences. Kelly argues that an individual is constantly seeking to improve their constructs by replacing old ones in the light of new experiences, and this, in turn, increases their repertory. Many construction systems can be widely shared while others are more personal. Kelly's theory is guided by a fundamental postulate and elaborated by means of eleven corollaries which are listed and briefly explained in Appendix 1. The corollaries follow from the postulate and are propositions which introduce types of construing and possible effects of replicated experience (Kelly, p35).

There are contentious views in the literature relating to the philosophical origins of Kelly's Personal Construct Theory (PCT). Ashworth (1981) argues that Kelly's theory is incoherent because of its parallels to phenomenology and its presuppositions which involve intentionality of consciousness and of action, yet elsewhere containing formal statements of positivism. Holland (1970), Keen (1975) and Wetherick (1970) however, see Kelly's PCT as being unproblematically phenomenological. It emphasises the personal viewpoint of the individual and Keen argues that constructs constitute a person's 'map of the lifeworld'. In this study I have used the complementary theories of Kelly and Heidegger to promote my understanding and interpretation of the students' stories. This integration may well be repugnant to the 'expert' philosopher and strategist, but it may be that my study will stimulate discussion and debate. Neimeyer and Neimeyer (1985) contend that provocative contributions often steer debate away from the stereotypical utilisation of theories and thereby present new and challenging ways of thinking about them.

Keen (1975) claims that Kelly's approach is essentially phenomenological because of its acceptance of personal experience as an essential domain, yet Bolton (1979) refutes the links between PCT and phenomenology on the grounds that it is essentially subjectivist and not directly focused upon the lived experience. Kelly himself claimed in his early work that PCT and phenomenology had no affiliation –

> we cannot consider the psychology of personal constructs a phenomenological theory, if that means ignoring the personal construction of the psychologist who does the observing.

(Kelly, p174)

But, this quote appears to be referring to Husserlian phenomenology and the concept of bracketing as explored earlier in this chapter, rather than Heidegger's hermeneutic phenomenology. In addition, I am not using PCT as a psychologist or in the belief that it is a phenomenological theory, I am using it to demonstrate the students' constructs emerging and changing over time. It is significant that ten of the eleven corollaries which Kelly uses as the basis of his construct theory, make specific reference to the 'person' and yet traditional psychology is not, in the main, about persons.

Bannister and Fransella (1986, pp29-30) using the work of Kelly, define what a person is. I have presented Heidegger's concept of the person alongside Kelly's for comparison in Table 2.1. Essentially, the core of Kelly's statements refers to constructivism which asserts that individuals create their own understanding of the world and this in turn affects how they act in relation to this meaningful world. Personal Construct Theory supports the existentialist view that people are actively involved in making their own lives and decisions. Kelly aspires to phenomenological principles throughout his text and states;

> Suppose we begin by assuming that the fundamental thing about life is that it goes on. It isn't that something makes you go on; the going on is the thing itself. It isn't that motives make a man come alert and do things; his alertness is an aspect of his very being.

(Kelly, p85)

The basis of Kelly's PCT is 'Constructive Alternativism' which asserts that reality does not reveal itself to us directly, but rather is subject to as many different constructions as we are able to invent; any event is open to a variety of interpretations (Buckenham, 1998). Kelly however, is keen to state that constructive alternativism represents a philosophical point of view and not a philosophical system.

Elliston and McCormick (1977, p71) discuss 'imagining', 'remembering' and 'signifying' as concepts within phenomenology. These appear to resemble the components of what Kelly terms 'construing'. 'Imagining' may be the skill required to form a conceptual repertory which Kelly claims is developed through experience. 'Remembering' past events also assists an individual to construe or anticipate future events, and to assess the accuracy of that anticipation. The concept of 'signifying' in phenomenology, when related to PCT, is the form in which we choose to communicate our constructs. Those construction systems which can be communicated can be widely shared through public construction systems or symbolism and language. Constructs can 'work' for an individual and help to make sense and assist with operating in particular situations and environments. They

Table 2.1   Concept of the Person

Kelly	Heidegger
You are convinced of your own separateness from others, you rely on the privacy of your own consciousness.	Dasein depends upon private interpretation in order to comprehend everyday experiences.
You are convinced of the integrity of the completeness of your experience in that you believe that all parts of it are ultimately relateable because you are the experiencer.	Ontology is the priority of Dasein - that is, experience and discovery are related and are the driving forces of our being.
You are convinced of your own continuity over time; you believe that in a significant sense you are the same person as you were when you were a child, you possess your own biography and live in relation to it.	The term which Heidegger uses to describe such an entity is 'temporality' and this incorporates 'historicity' which is an appreciation of one's past, and 'potentiality' - an appreciation for what one might be in the future.
You are convinced that your actions are causal, that you have purposes, that you intend and thereby accept a partial responsibility for the effects of what you do.	The person exists only in the performance of intentional acts and this is what distinguishes people from objects.
You are convinced of the separate existence of other persons by analogy with yourself, you assume a comparability of subjective experience between yourself and others.	Recognition that people are separate entities even though we encounter each other on a daily basis. He states; "the world is always the one I share with others" (p155) and by so doing, experiences are shared.

may also be considered as hypotheses through which individuals test their world. But, in order to function within their environment, each individual acts within the limits allowed by their construct system, which implies some form of structure and organisation of constructs, so that activation of one kind of construct may well activate related others. However, Kelly recognises that a person may not necessarily be able to articulate the constructions she/he places upon their world ; "Some of his [sic] constructions are not symbolised in words, he can only express them in pantomime" (Kelly, p12). In other words, Kelly is receptive to various ways of obtaining and interpreting meaning associated with peoples' constructs - a similar tolerance as Heidegger's hermeneutic philosophy.

Davidson (1986) also draws parallels between phenomenology and PCT in proposing that a person can sometimes gain or lose a belief, not by change of mind on that topic, but by revision on some other, which shifts the equilibrium. Kelly states that a person's constructs are open to revision or "outright abandonment" when their view of certain topics is modified in some way (Kelly, p30). Further, Elliston and McCormick (1977) describe 'intentionality' as a primal striving within phenomenology which implies conceptual representational functions similar to Kelly's 'fundamental postulate'. If 'intentionality' refers to the mind's directedness within a phenomenological tradition, this must surely equate to the fundamental postulate which states that "a person's processes are psychologically chanellised by the ways he [sic] anticipates events"? (Kelly, p32).

Although there are many similar concepts in PCT that do not constitute a breach with phenomenology, there is one aspect of the theory which is distinct from it. That is, PCT requires that there be an inner mental system of constructs which might give the impression that the outer world is meaningless, physical stimulation. I think the theory is couched generally in phenomenological terms and thereby extinguishes all temptation to associate it with objective methods and systems of enquiry. I have used a modified grid and the theory of personal constructs to make sense of data from students within a hermeneutic phenomenological framework. PCT has lent itself to this order and I have no qualms in defending its use within this framework. Kelly himself hoped that the theory would be used in many varied contexts.

Summary

This chapter has attempted to offer a rationale for the choices made in establishing the philosophical foundations of the study. The reader has been introduced to the guiding perspectives and special terminology used within the text and the importance of the underlying principles of ontology, hermeneutic phenomenology and PCT. I have related Heideggerian phenomenology to the work of nurse theorists which I hope will provide some familiarity with the theoretical base. Care and concern, the central tenets of Heidegger's hermeneutics have been explored in relation to nursing theory and, finally, Kelly's PCT has been associated with phenomenology to explain why it has been particularly useful in this study. I hope to have made explicit the relationships and congruencies between ontology, hermeneutics and PCT.

In the next chapter, the methods and techniques used to collect and analyse data are described and justified. In it I intend to illuminate formal and informal research processes, demonstrate the use of methods and techniques in the practical setting and share some of my reflections upon these with the reader.

3 Methodology - Processes, Praxis and Ponderances

The previous chapter described how Ontology, Heideggerian Hermeneutic Phenomenology and Kelly's Personal Construct Theory provided a philosophical basis for my research. The chapter focused upon the congruency between these three perspectives and the contribution they have made toward my understanding of the data gathered. This chapter takes the reader along the decision trail associated with the methodology.

In order to portray the evolutionary and dynamic processes of data collection and analysis in this study, I intend to present the rationale for choice of method or technique used to collect data, the processes involved in utilising these in practice and my reflections on these methods and techniques following my experiences. The methodology will be presented in a sequential fashion, as activities evolved in response to the needs of the investigation and dictated by the development of students throughout the Diploma of Higher Education in Nursing Studies course. Some of the events occurred through serendipity, having not been anticipated or planned and yet transpired as being the most effective and illuminating aspects of the research process.

Van Manen (1990) advocates innovation in phenomenological research and attention by researchers to 'personal signature' which characterises human science research and emphasises the strengths of the research and the researcher. Phenomenologists often use literary sources such as poetry, novels and stories and aesthetic sources such as role play, opera and art to portray lifeworld and give expression to the lived experience of their subjects. Early in this study I recognised the need to be more creative and flexible in my approach to data collection. It became apparent during the second contact phase with students that they needed a more open forum to allow them to consider what was happening to them during the Course, reflect upon these events and to verbalise these experiences to me. I anticipated that standard methods such as interviews and questionnaires would be too rigid and as a consequence, students' expressions and descriptions of experiences might be restricted. The methodology required to satisfy such an agenda

39

presented me with a challenge. Working within a hermeneutic phenomenological approach, I was conscious of certain philosophical and processual demands such as respecting unique experiences; identifying commonalities between students; inclusion of my own experience and the effects of this upon the data and consideration of activities associated with the hermeneutic circle. In addition, I was aware of the license that phenomenology gives to the researcher; the freedom to be creative and respond to situations occurring.

I considered the data collection methods and techniques used in this study to be evolutionary because each set of data acted as a signpost for, or a determinant of, the following data collection phase. Subsequent methods were not developed until I had absorbed the essence of students' experiences and identified the best way to capture their ongoing development. Each method enabled students to address key issues raised in previous phases and allowed constructs to be identified. The phases were analogous to a signpost because they offered me direction and represented the different journeys; the 'becoming' journey for the students and my own hermeneutic journey.

Table 3.1 provides an overview of the data collection phases throughout the study.

Ethical considerations

Ethical aspects of phenomenological research are particularly important because of the place of the researcher as interpreter of the lifeworld of others and as recipient of potentially exposing information. These issues have been discussed in the nursing research literature (Haggman-Laitila, 1999; Seymour and Ingleton, 1999; Usher and Holmes, 1997). To address this potential problem in the study, participants were offered opportunities [in accordance with the reflexive nature of phenomenological research] to respond to my interpretations, and to make additions and corrections at each stage of the research.

The potential for criticism of perceived bias in qualitative research, by those adopting more traditional approaches, may be fuelled by the realisation that the study is always linked to the person of the researcher; the consequence being, that an individual study cannot be repeated in the same form by another researcher (Haggman-Laitila, 1999). Perceived investigator bias is discussed by Denzin and Lincoln (1994) but Christman et al. (1995) indicate the variety of ways in which individual researchers approach the same research and outline the contribution of their unique perspectives upon the processes. Indeed,

40

Table 3.1   Significant Dates

Feb 1992	'Project 2000' commenced in the study area
Feb 1994	Study cohort commenced
Feb 1994	Questionnaires to total student cohort in College (n=56, 100%)
Aug 1994	One-to-one interviews with 8 participants
Nov 1994 - Apr 1995	Nine focus group interviews with tutors in College (n=27, 100%)
Feb 1995	Repertory grid technique with 8 participants in College
Aug 1995	Present tense commentary with 8 participants in College or the participants' homes
Jan - Mar 1996	One-to-one interviews with practitioners in their own work areas (n=15)
Jun 1996	Student participants (n=8) submitted reflective practice portfolios
Sep 1996	The 'College of Health' became part of the 'Faculty of Health and Social Care' within the University
Nov 1996	Student participants wrote their letters (n=7, 87%)
Feb 1997	Questionnaires to student cohort in College (n=28, 100%)
Feb 1997	Study cohort completed the Course

Lamb and Huttlinger (1989) argue that 'investigator bias' is a resource for qualitative researchers, acting as a guide to data gathering, creativity and for understanding interpretations. Reflexivity is seen as central to the avoidance of the researcher forming too superficial a picture of participants which could misrepresent the individual.

In addition, I have made efforts to thoroughly describe and justify my decision trail throughout this chapter, in order to clarify the authenticity and ethical standards of the research.

Similarly to May (1991), I acknowledge that the methods I used to collect data from my student participants stimulated self-reflection, reappraisal and in some instances, catharsis. Methods which were liable to provoke such a level of disclosure had to be thoroughly planned and considered and I achieved this through discussions with my supervisors and colleagues.

In order to establish a sense of trust with my participants, I strove to address issues of perceived power imbalance between the students and myself as a senior lecturer and researcher. My title within the educational establishment could have been somewhat formidable to students at the outset of the Course. I was aware of this and made efforts to be open and honest in answering questions about the research and the potential effects upon them as student's on the Course. Each time I met with them to ask for their co-operation with data collection I was aware of the power dimension and ensured that they had opportunity to withdraw from the study without retribution either from me or from the institution. Feminist theorists have been sensitive to power issues and relationships in fieldwork and expose the problems associated with such power discrepancies (Stacey, 1988). Ramos (1989) recognises the need for a more balanced relationship as being the key to meaningful data collection in phenomenological research, where the intimacy and intensity of relationships is central to interpretation.

Usher and Arthur (1998) argue that obtaining informed consent is not a static 'once and for all' event, but an active, dynamic process of renegotiation between the researcher and the participant. It may be that I should have asked more formally for students' consent to participate at each data collection phase.

My participants shared personal stories which, had they been 'leaked', could have caused problems amongst them. However, they trusted me not to tell anyone; I was acutely aware that to do so would have breached their confidence, could have caused tension between participants and induced withdrawal from the study. I was also aware of my responsibility as a role model from both a nursing and research perspective that to divulge confidential information would be considered unprofessional behaviour. It is a professional expectation that nurses engage in ethical conduct; indeed, students are taught the importance of the moral nature of the nurse-patient/client relationship from the outset of the Course (Smith, 1996).

During the three years of data collection in which I was taken into the students' private social and experiential world, our relationship developed to such an extent that I found great difficulty divorcing their personalities from their names. Throughout the analysis stages I continued to use the names of the students to avoid confusion for me as the analyst and interpreter. Although the students agreed for me to use their names in the final draft of the thesis, I chose to override this permission in view of potential long term ethical implications. All names of participants in this study have, therefore, been replaced by pseudonyms. However, the extent to which anonymity is achieved may depend upon the motive of the reader and their knowledge of the particular study area.

The students and I discussed the possibility of using the data for other purposes such as publications and conference papers and they agreed that this would be acceptable, providing I shared my intentions prior to submission.

[It should also be noted that I had sought approval from the Principal of the College of Health at the same time I submitted a proposal to the Research Degrees Committee at the institution with whom I registered.]

The specific implications of the study for students, practitioners, tutors and myself are acknowledged throughout the methodology as I describe and justify the methods and techniques used. I believe that by doing this, the implications remain context-bound and pertinent to each stage of the research process, rather than divorced from the situations from which they arise.

Embarkation - the starting point

An open-ended questionnaire, consisting of four questions, designed to generate opinion/perception-related answers was distributed to all students in the cohort (N=56) within the first three weeks of the Course. This was seen to be an appropriate time, prior to the theory aspect of the Course commencing and before exposure to clinical placements. Questions tapped perceptions of nursing and expectations of the Course and what students believed they had to offer nursing [Appendix 2].

I accessed the group after a lecture in college, introduced myself and gave an explanation of my intentions for the study and possible outcomes. This first encounter with the students enabled me to engage people in the study and determine their level of interest. The main aim of the questionnaire was to gain insight into perceptions and the level of understanding about nursing and this sensitised me to possible lines of enquiry for the next data collection phase. Blumer (1954) suggests that exposure to key issues sometimes assists the researcher to identify the direction of questioning. The questionnaire data certainly provided a starting point and stimulated my thoughts. Subsequently it occurred to me that key issues identified at this early stage were provisional, became unstable as the study progressed and more orientated to the individual. All students completed the questionnaire and the data were analysed using a simple thematic method to determine key issues that had significance for the student group.

The student volunteers

After the questionnaire was completed by the cohort of students, ten volunteers agreed to participate. However, one student did not arrive at a later date for the first one-to-one interview and I took this to mean that she no longer wanted to be included in the sample. Another student left early in the Course but was interviewed later as a course leaver. The remaining eight students continued to participate in the study until they qualified three years later.

I explained to the original ten students about my interest in them and how I intended to follow their progress through the Common Foundation Programme. This was before I transferred to PhD and the potential for the study had yet to be realised. They seemed quite excited by the prospect of being 'special' in the group but were anxious about my expectation of them. I reassured them that they could opt out of the study at any time without any repercussions on their progress through the Course.

I approached the Academic Manager to suggest that I had no 'personal' students in this particular cohort, as to do so may complicate my role as researcher. My only other contact with the student group was as a teacher delivering a research awareness module in the Common Foundation Programme. The assessment strategy for that module was a timed exam paper which meant that all papers were anonymised and my role as a teacher had no bearing upon the participants in the study.

I had also considered that paying particular attention to a few students in a cohort might stir some resentment in the group as a whole

44

and I wanted to ensure that this could not be exacerbated and impinge on the quality of teaching or supervision they received. With such a small sample, I was unable to assure confidentiality as experiences might be identified in the data as belonging to one person or another, particularly as the other students in the group had seen the participants volunteer. Students understood that this might be so and agreed that they would receive transcripts of all interactions between me and each individual. They could then decide if there were certain parts of their data that they would wish to have removed and also verify that my recording of the interactions were accurate. I also gave each of the participants a detailed summary of my impressions of their development and changing constructs at a late stage in the study. This gave them the opportunity to give additional comment and return the summaries amended.

Much of the data obtained through the questionnaires provided me with a baseline understanding for students' development and progression and contributed specifically to Chapter 6 'Intentionality - Comportment Toward Nursing and the Course'.

The realisation - one-to-one interviews

The themes elicited from the questionnaire data shaped the questions for the semi-structured interviews with the student participants (Appendix 3). I chose to interview the students, despite my claim that interviews are 'too rigid' because I felt confident with the method and hoped to engage them in conversation about themselves, nursing and their nurse education. The interviews served as a starting point to a more creative strategy.

The interviews occurred after students had completed six months of the Course. Dates were agreed in advance with students and their consent for the interviews to be tape recorded was gained prior to their arrival. The interviews were conducted in a small room in college and the conversation was initiated by asking the student to talk about themselves and in particular, what they were doing during the time leading up to commencement of the Course. All interviews were tape-recorded and the tapes, along with the transcript, became the material for subsequent interpretation of meaning. I made efforts to focus conversation upon the students' lifeworld and how they responded to the initial impressions of nursing and nurse education. I hoped that the interview would be a positive experience for the students and lay the foundation for a fruitful relationship between us during their attendance on the Course and beyond. All participants responded to questioning and

I was able to gain some insight into their previous lives which was useful throughout the study. The students' voice intonations and accents are so firmly engrained in my psyche, that a mention of any of their names brings a flood of memorable quotations in dialect to the fore.

It was during initial analysis of these interviews that a change in students' constructs became apparent; and these early constructs are portrayed in Chapter 6. Growth of perceptions and shifting emphases had occurred as a result of completing six months of the Course, and this intrigued me. In order to capture the essence of experiences, which served as a catalyst for development, I realised that I would need to use approaches to data collection which enabled flexibility so that students could portray their changing perceptions on paper as well as verbally. This realisation led to some serious consideration of options, the purpose of the study, possible outcomes, my ability to proceed within a developing framework and possible implications for the students and the study, of allowing the study to develop beyond the original remit. I found this particular phase of the study stimulating and exciting and the prospect of its development demanded a greater commitment from me and the students. I met with them to discuss possible ways to advance and improve the quality of data which would enable me to gain a more comprehensive understanding of their perspective.

Although I had intended from the outset that this study would be qualitative in nature I had been uncertain, during this phase, of the philosophical origins and theoretical underpinnings of the study. This has already been discussed in Chapter 2, but it was at this stage, six months after the students had started the Course, that I realised the importance of selecting methods which embraced the philosophical orientation of my study. Implicit in the integrity of the study must be a commitment to methods and techniques which satisfy the fundamental concepts of phenomenology. I developed a criterion which guided me throughout the remainder of the research and to which I referred as the core of good practice for research using this approach. I wanted my participants to have the freedom to illuminate their personal experience while I would use my professional experience and reflections to help me understand their horizon. I believed that reflection-on-action (Schon, 1987) should be central to students' processes of remembering and conveying experiences to me. Using reflective skills prepared the students for other aspects of the Course which advantaged them in some small way. It meant that they had had experience of formally reflecting before other students in their cohort were required to do so.

I considered the importance of enabling a power shift from me, as a senior lecturer, to the students, so that they could govern the pace and level of disclosure. I felt enlightened and satisfied with these changes and began planning a strategy which would fulfil this criterion.

RepGrid - accessing constructions

Repertory Grid Technique (RepGrid) and its underlying philosophy, Personal Construct Theory (PCT), have been used in nursing research to identify nurses' self perceptions of caring (Morrison, 1990), contributions of nursing, midwifery and health visiting to the therapeutic milieu (Scholes and Freeman, 1994), as a clinical tool to document information from clients (Pollock, 1986), as an approach to the socialisation of nurse trainees (Heyman, Shaw and Harding, 1983), to examine nurses' feelings about patients with feeding needs (Barnes, 1990) and as a way of analysing the feelings nurses experience in clinical practice (White, 1996). All these studies except Morrison, used the grid technique quantitatively; that is, researchers measured changing constructs of their subjects. In this way, grids enable constructs to develop hierarchically and the intention is to discover subsystems. Morrison (1991; 1990) explored nurses' perceptions of the concept of caring. His respondents were asked to identify likenesses and differences between elements in a grid and from these, bi-polar constructs were determined. He used a category scheme to organise the 200 constructs collected which were then reduced to a seven category framework. He claims that this provided a detailed picture of caring and nursing practice. However, the elements which students had to comment upon, were chosen by the researcher, rather than the students themselves and in my view this is a weakness in Morrison's study.

Scholes and Freeman (1994) developed an approach using reflective dialogue and repertory grids to explore the meaning of practice to the practitioner.

> Facilitating the expression of change enabled the participants to confer meaning on their own circumstances and to deliberately review their own personal progression and experience of transition.
>
> (Scholes and Freeman, 1994, p888)

These authors used reflection and RepGrid in symbiosis which enabled them to examine changes in meaning. The analytical process of reflection captured transitional activities of thought which demonstrate personal and professional change encountered over a period of time.

This can then be compared to data from the grid which also captures alterations in perceptions. This study inspired me to consider how I could use RepGrid to capture my participants' changing perceptions and constructions of nursing during the first year of their nurse education programme.

Rawlinson (1995) reviews the use of RepGrids in studies of nurses and social workers and includes, within this critique, comments about socialisation studies such as Davis (1983), Heyman et al. (1983), and Wilkinson (1982). From these studies he draws conclusions and chooses to caution readers about divorcing the technique from the theory of personal constructs [which many do], simply because the use of grids appears attractive as a method. During development of the repertory grid technique and a complete theory of personality, Kelly (1955) promoted the use of the technique separately from the theory (Thomas and Harri-Augstein, 1985), or combined with the theoretical approach (Button, 1985). Construct theory was originally stated in very abstract terms so that it could be applied to any culture and at any time. Kelly designed the theory with a wide range of convenience that therefore should not be tied to any single concept-phenomenon. Fransella and Bannister (1977, p4) comment that it is the user of the theory who has to supply a context in which the theory might make sense.

To develop the grid technique into a method congruent with phenomenological principles all students' statements, relevant to the aims of the study, were extracted from the transcripts of the one-to-one interviews of the previous data set. The individual statements were organised on a unique grid for each student in order to accommodate comment from students regarding their perception of the statement at the time they said it [six months into the Course], their perception at the time of the RepGrid exercise [one year into the Course], and how they thought they would perceive the statement as qualified nurses.

Kelly's theory of personal constructs proposes that people create their meanings of the world through existing cognitive constructs and, in so doing, link old knowledge with new knowledge and this was evident in the grid data. The following are typical of many examples;

I thought I had experience of just about everything. I now see that I hadn't. I'm experiencing new things every time I go on a placement.

(Sarah, RepGrid)

Until recently ... I thought psychology etc was a complete and utter waste of time. I don't think I was using it. I was sitting there thinking

48

"what good is this going to be while I'm making beds on the wards?"
But when I'm out in the community ... I was sitting there and I was
coming out with these sociological comments about the sick role. I
thought ... this wasn't me. I didn't realise that any of it was going in or
doing any good ... but it was there.

(Ben, RepGrid)

I said that being a nursing auxiliary had helped me with basic skills;
bed making and washing patients. Now the experience has given me
more confidence when I'm on the ward. When I'm qualified, I will have
the knowledge to help other auxiliaries, because I'll know what they're
going through.

(Marie, RepGrid)

Evidence of shift in perceptions was often accompanied by a change of construct associated with understanding the role and nature of nurses and nursing.

In many PCT studies a typical grid has an 'emergent pole' and a 'contrast pole' which enables researchers to measure the distance travelled in terms of constructions. The function of viewing constructs as bi-polar is so that it can be mathematically represented. As this was not the intention of the grid in this study, I chose to use an emergent pole - 'Myself as I was' and a desired pole 'Myself as a qualified nurse'. This demanded skills of reflection and forecasting from the students in order to assess how they had already changed and anticipated changing as they progressed into the qualified nurse role. I tape recorded all the RepGrid encounters and transcribed these verbatim. Transcripts were given to the students to seek verification and authenticity. Both the grids and the transcripts were used during the analysis stage as one complemented the other. Although students had written on the grid, the detailed explanations of what they had written and why, captured on tape, were of paramount importance during the analytical stage. In addition to transcribing the RepGrid encounter, I also wrote notes alongside the transcript relating to the corollaries [a discussion of how the corollaries in personal construct theory relate to phenomenology and apply to the data from this phase has been offered in Chapter 2]. Part of the process for analysis of these data involved separating all the statements for each individual student and assigning the statement to the different corollaries. For example, under the heading 'Sociality Corollary' Clare had the following statements -

I felt really shy in the large group. Now I speak out more.
I think people have a different attitude to you when you have a uniform on.
I felt like a spare part and really awkward at placements.

(Clare, RepGrid)

This corollary enabled me to identify the social processes involved in 'being a student' and their perceptions of their clinical colleagues and peers and how they felt they were 'fitting in' to various groups encountered.

My reflections and thoughts after using the method constitute several thousand words written soon after this data collection phase. In order to present a flavour of my learning associated with using the method I have chosen to paraphrase my reflections here [Dictaphone, Feb. 1995].

This method is less formal than a traditional interview and takes on a more conversational style. Having said that, there is a huge imbalance between researcher and participant talk time. The transcripts show at least 90% of talk is in the students' voice. The method really enabled the students to tell stories and they injected a substantial amount of humour into the explanations. Afterwards, they said they had enjoyed using the grids and talking about their development. The students were in control of their information and the pace and I found this comforting and engaging. Some students were able to reflect better than others and some were better at forecasting how they would feel as qualified nurses. All students commented on 'Myself as I am now' although this appears to be an unstable aspect of the grid. Students have said that things could change over a period of days depending on how they were feeling. The 'Myself as I am now' should be recognised as a snapshot, rather than indicative of a longer period of time. Eye to eye contact has been difficult to sustain at times because it is necessary to sit beside the student and work through the grid. The grid becomes the focus of the encounter and to some extent, appears to be less threatening and embarrassing for the students. The tape was much more difficult to transcribe than the one-to-one interviews because both the researcher and the participant refer to the grid in conversation. I recognised that I may not 'keep up' with the development of the conversation and deliberately interjected at times to record on tape what we were referring to on the grid. Students reported a therapeutic value to completing the grid and the encounter which enabled them to see how far they had progressed from a personal and professional perspective. Interestingly, they often didn't make the comments I had anticipated. This demonstrates our contrasting frames of reference and will be important to recognise and address in future data collection phases. There is a need to be totally student led so that my misinterpretations do not cloud the students' meanings of their experiences. I am pleased that I gave the students the grids a week prior to meeting with them. It enabled them to take time to reflect and fill in the grid. Using statements from the one-to-one interviews as elements on the grid meant that the importance of the statements (or unimportance) was validated at the RepGrid encounter. Some of the statements were glossed over and this indicated to me that what they had talked about in the previous data phase was no longer of any importance. It is imperative that the encounter is tape recorded and transcribed so that the researcher retains the elaborations and explanations for purposes of analysis.

The RepGrid data collection phase served the purpose of enabling the students to develop insights into the changes occurring within them, both professionally and personally. Initial analysis of the RepGrid data suggested that students often had significant experiences which could be associated with shifts of understanding and professional growth. Denzin (1989) refers to these types of experiences as "epiphanies", where individual character is revealed during the event. Various strategies were considered at this stage which would enable these epiphanies to be captured with the intention of analysing their essence and meaning. Using hermeneutics, it is also expected that researchers approach the data from an informed perspective and develop interpretations and understandings enlightened by their own experience (Packer and Addison, 1989).

Crotty (1996) argues for recognising the individual as a conscious agent who is the most knowledgeable expert on his or her life and that they should be enabled to tell their experiences as they have been lived. I thought it was imperative that my participants were permitted to tell their own story in their own words and in response to their own reflections on the experience over time. In order to achieve this, I developed a technique based on an original idea by Witkin (1994) who reported using commentary on relived events in a social science study.

51

Present tense commentary - sharing experiences

Many authors discuss the benefits of using storytelling as a powerful vehicle for communication, education and preservation of cultural identity (Bowles, 1995; Boykin and Schoenhofer, 1991; Fairbairn, 1993). Narrative is also recognised as a valuable tool in qualitative research (Helling, 1988; Labor and Waletzky, 1966; Sandelowski, 1991). Some parallels can be drawn between these methods and present tense commentary, although the main differences are the use of reflection-on-action and the purpose of the method.

The full process of using present tense commentary is explained in Mitchell (1999), but I shall present the basic process of conducting the technique and main issues here.

Prior to using the technique I considered a number of issues with regard to the training of participants, support systems for the participants and myself, and subsequent data collection phases. Participants had the process fully explained to them so that they understood the value of the technique and what to expect. The technique involved getting the students to relive events and simulate the encounters that had actually occurred in their clinical practice or college environment through commentary in the present tense.

I compiled written guidelines (Appendix 4) for the students about the types of experiences they might wish to recall and they were supplied with an example and a model for structured reflection (Johns, 1996). I thought that structured reflection might assist with recalling the experience and enable the student to give additional information about his/her performance as part of the commentary. This might give me an insight into the students' perceptions of their development during the two years on the Course thus far. Dates were agreed with students to meet with me, with their written reflections, to convey their chosen experiences as commentary. The commentaries were tape recorded and transcripts were returned to the students for authentication. Immediately after the commentaries, I often felt that students had 'dumped' their baggage on me and I had to decide how I could make best use of my feelings. I decided to write summaries and found this to be cathartic, allowing me to lay to rest some of the stirred emotions which occurred as a result of listening to the stories. It also enabled me to think about students' development and why these changes might be occurring. The summaries also contributed to my analysis and identification of my own 'emerging Selves' (Chapter 5).

The selection of events and construction of the commentary proceeded freely under the control of the students with minimum interference from me. This was seen to be congruent with a hermeneutic phenomenological approach. Witkin (1994) acknowledges that this type of technique can be refreshing and enjoyable for participants, but that it can also be a time of heightened anxiety concerning the degree of self exposure involved.

I felt I needed to be prepared for any eventualities, and with this in mind I asked a colleague with advanced counselling skills to be available for the students. I thought it would be inappropriate for me to take on a counselling role as becoming therapeutically involved with the students might have compromised the students' development. It transpired that counselling services were not required by any of the students, although there were many emotional accounts shared.

Students described some of the most powerful and meaningful events in their practice, but referred to them as everyday events, when they were 'just there'. They were there for patients and their families at times when intimacy through touch and words were shared. The students talked of feeling 'undervalued', 'unsupported', 'bemused', and 'frustrated' with the reality of clinical practice. In all recalled events there was evidence of enormous giving of themselves, commitment and personal and professional development; traits which the students themselves identified. Much of this data contributed toward the development of Chapters 7 and 8 concerned with 'Thrownness' and 'Being-in-the-world-with-others'. Becoming a nurse was expressed through experiences where they felt comfortable, accepted, confident, competent and those which gave them a sense of belonging. These stories were contrasted with others where students felt uncomfortable, rejected, in conflict with their beliefs, unsure and incompetent.

The main attraction of this technique is that it positions the Self of the teller centrally in the narrative given. It is literally a story of, and about, the Self in relation to an experience on the Self. It is also through the special nature of present tense commentary that I came to an understanding of the students' position because of my similar personal experiences. Indeed, during some of the commentaries, both the student and I became emotionally touched by the strength and richness of the description.

Because of the investment of energy in this technique, I warned students that they should stop the commentary immediately if they became uncomfortable or felt that there was something they did not want to say. At the outset, students were given the opportunity to choose the experiences on which they were going to reflect and convey to me. They need not have chosen emotionally loaded experiences if they preferred not to relive these particular events, but I needed to consider the possibility that the technique itself might coax them into a vulnerable position through which more intimate details could be elicited than they wished to provide.

With hindsight, the process of conducting the present tense commentaries, although involved, was successful and the technique yielded very rich data. I learned a great deal about researcher sensitivity and considerations necessary prior to using such a technique.

There were some negative aspects to using this type of commentary, not least that the skills of conveying the story and the skills involved in reflection-on-action, without doubt, added to the students' workload. However, they reported benefit from having experience of reflection prior to using it for their next Course assignment which involved reflecting on events in practice and analysing them.

Students' analysis of their own development - reflective practice portfolios

At the time that this study was conducted, students on the Diploma of HE in Nursing Studies courses were required to submit a 6000 word reflective practice portfolio as an assignment three months prior to completing the Course. Using a reflective model to assist reflection-on-action, students recorded three experiences related to a nursing issue, a teaching experience and a management issue from their clinical practice.

The students analysed these experiences to reveal professional development through analysis of action, decision making, identifying alternatives and reconsidering action for future practice. Wong, Kember, Chung and Yan (1995) express support for using reflection as a way of learning which facilitates the integration of theory with practice. It also provides the opportunity to turn every experience into a new potential learning experience. I believed that the reflective practice portfolios, as a method, would be congruent with a hermeneutic phenomenological approach for two reasons. Firstly because the central point to reflection is experience, which concurs with Heidegger's explanations of ontology having a main concern of understanding and giving meaning to experience, and secondly, because hermeneutic enquiry primarily focuses upon texts and how they are produced.

I seized this opportunity to utilise the students' reflective practice portfolios in order to discover the meanings that the selected events had for them. Understanding the context in which these events occurred was also important as it provided an 'historical consciousness' (Gadamer, 1977) essential to interpretation. This is seen to result in a fusion of the 'text-and-its-context' with the 'researcher-and-her-context'. Also, utilising their assignments at this stage in the Course, meant that I was not making any additional demands upon the students during a time when they felt particularly pressurised, coming up to completion of the Course.

The study participants all agreed willingly for me to use their portfolios as a method and furnished me with copies of their disks. I had no part in the marking of these portfolios which meant that I was released from 'myself as educationalist' and given the freedom to become 'myself as researcher' whilst analysing them.

The experiences captured in the reflective practice portfolios demonstrated professional growth of the study participants, in particular the ways in which they would deal with situations which had previously caused them concern. Some of the data from this phase has been used in Chapter 10 concerned with being an 'active subject'. It is concerned with the development of skills which enable students to act autonomously in anticipation of, or to, events in practice.

Severing ties - a few final questions

After this episode of data collection and through the analysis, it became apparent that the students were progressing on their journey from layperson to nurse. I thought that a final one-to-one interview would be appropriate to discuss outstanding issues with them and to provide a final validity check of their experiences. Personally, I needed to draw the study to an end. I also needed to acknowledge the remainder of the cohort who had contributed to initial data through the questionnaire distributed three years earlier. I managed to arrange a session with the whole group during their last week of attendance in college to give them some feedback on how the study was progressing and changes which had evolved during the three years. Without divulging too much about the participants [their peers], or the tentative findings at this stage, I gave indications about the direction and potential outcomes of the study. I did not link experiences to the relevant students, but I was able to demonstrate my main interpretations of what it had been like becoming a nurse for the participants in very general terms.

The students were amused that they had completed their Course in three years and yet it was likely that I would have another three years of study to endure. However, they showed a genuine empathy for my situation and willingly completed a questionnaire which, in addition to providing data, acted as a symbol of severance from the study.

My eight key participants were in the midst of the larger group and also completed the questionnaires. The questions were broadly framed (Appendix 6) and provided students with the opportunity to reflect upon their development through the Course and factors which they perceived affected their transition and how they were feeling about undertaking the responsibilities of a qualified nurse.

By eliciting these additional data from other students in the cohort, I was able to compare and contrast answers from the questionnaire with those from my study participants. Similarities in responses were evident, even though experiences would have been unique to individuals. I also acknowledge that my eight participants would have been more attuned to particular issues than their counterparts in the cohort as a result of participating in the study.

At the end of this feedback session, my study participants stayed behind and requested that I keep in touch with them. They promised to write and inform me of their career developments. Time had almost elapsed and I had not arranged final one-to-one interviews with them. I felt that I had not been thorough enough in my severance from these particular eight individuals. The questionnaire had been an opportunity to gain data from the cohort but I felt it was inappropriate and an inadequate means of providing each of the key actors in this research with the opportunity to express their feelings associated with their departure. All my participants had successfully completed the Course and had secured staff nurse posts; most of them outside the study location. If I was to access them one last time, I needed to make decisions regarding the method quite quickly, whilst respecting the principles of the approach and with the intention of continuing the evolutionary nature of the data. I returned to the hermeneutic phenomenological literature that I had accumulated during the three years to search for inspiration.

"This is how it was for me" - summarising the journey in a letter

> I also write because I think one must not only share what one thinks, or the conclusions one has reached, but one must also share to help others reach their conclusions.
>
> (Vezeau, 1993)

The development of aesthetic knowledge in nursing has been encouraged by several authors (Benner and Wrubel, 1989; Carper, 1978;

Watson, 1985; Wolfer, 1993; Younger, 1990). Support is given to the concept that there is a need for nursing as a profession that cares for individuals to develop methods and techniques in enquiry which utilise aesthetic knowing of an individual's situations and experiences. Similarly, researchers (Eisner and Peshkin, 1990; Sandelowski, 1991; van Manen, 1990) provide strong arguments for the utilisation of aesthetic methods and processes in qualitative research which illuminate lived experience. Appleton (1991), Chinn and Watson (1994), Cumbie and Rutherford (1994), Valle and Halling (1989) and Vezeau (1992) all recognise the potential for exploring the breadth and depth of human experience using non-conventional means of collecting data. As a result of exploring these issues and considering my options, the potential for letter writing as a data collection technique was explored and developed.

I managed to access all eight participants during their last days in the study location in their various clinical placements and provided them with guidelines (Appendix 7) and a final request to provide data through a letter, for the study. I thought that communication through a letter would provide a mutual world where the reader and the teller could meet to share the realities of experience and yet use simple language instead of technical jargon. I expected that the correspondence would be chatty and anecdotal and provide a departure point - an opportunity for student catharsis related to their Course on paper and also a means whereby loose ends could be tied up. Within the guidelines, students were asked to write to a friend [real or fictional], who they had not seen for at least three years, outlining pertinent details relating to decisions taken and significant experiences which contributed to becoming a nurse. This was seen to be an appropriate way of completing the data collection for the study and for students to be released from it.

The letters to a real or fictional friend were accompanied by an additional letter to me, from the students, wishing me success with my study and hoping that their attached letters would be useful data. These letters arrived up to eight weeks after completion of the Course - a couple had forgotten about the letters in the excitement of terminating their student contracts and commencing new posts as staff nurses. Data collected through this method contributed, in the main, to chapters within Part IV, and especially to the poems which conclude the part.

All letters to me included the students' new addresses and I anticipated that we would meet sometime in the future, an expectation which was fulfilled when I was invited to present this total student cohort at a ceremony to the Chancellor of the University for their Diploma awards some ten months after they had completed the Course. This acted as the real termination of our journeys together. I presented each of them by name and they received their Diplomas of Higher Education in Nursing Studies awards in the local cathedral.

It should be noted that the methods and techniques described here as evolutionary and directional required less and less involvement from me as students were empowered to portray their lifeworlds according to their own and not my agenda.

Recordings of my reflections on the processes

Throughout this study, I have endeavoured to keep notes of my feelings, reflections, observations and learning. For ease, much of this has been recorded on a dictaphone. I find it distracting when I have to find a pen and paper when I have ideas. It has been much easier to pick up the dictaphone, press a button and speak.

Transcribing my recordings has been an interesting exercise. I always ensured that the dates and times of my utterances were recorded first and then continued with whatever I wanted to say. Most of these occurred after data collection phases or when I had ideas relating to methods or when I just wanted to say something relevant about any of the study participants. The dictaphone became an extension of me, as is my work diary. When I came to transcribe the recordings I was surprised to hear many modes of the same voice. Driving along the motorway between university sites, I have a raised tone with staccato diction against an auditory backdrop of the car engine and road noise. My sentence construction is poor as I try to concentrate on the traffic as well as what I need to record. I am fearful of losing my thread of thought, or dread the passing thought disappearing completely. Another common voice on the dictaphone is that of my sleepy mumblings which occur in the middle of the night. Sometimes I do not remember recording anything overnight, but the evidence is on the tape the next morning and what I have recorded is usually associated with my reading or writing the evening before. More commonly is a desperate voice, eager to record something I had not anticipated or thought of before. There is an air of excitement in the tone and recognition of the potential of an idea.

These recordings remind me of my mood and capture the essence of my learning. Although many of my reflections have not been used directly in this thesis, they have served a very useful role within the hermeneutic circle; mainly to help clarify the circularity of understanding occurring between the data, the students and myself. I have been able to reflect on how I felt at times during the research process and what has inspired and demotivated me. I have also found the tapes useful to remind me that I am responsible for contributing to the data as a participant.

Considerations for hermeneutic analysis

The purpose of data analysis in phenomenology is to;

> preserve the uniqueness of each lived experience of the phenomenon while permitting an understanding of the meaning of the phenomenon itself.
>
> (Banonis, 1989, p168)

Beck (1994), Koch (1995), Nelms (1996), Omery (1983), Walters (1995) and Wilson and Hutchinson (1991) present a variety of frameworks available for the analysis of phenomenological data. These frameworks involve transcribing material, coding data into themes, clustering these into categories and forming a classification of attributes of the phenomena (Jasper, 1994). All these researchers discuss the analysis of interview data - none of them consider other data collection methods or techniques and I have found this particularly frustrating when all the phenomenological literature advocates the use of creative approaches.

The analytical process in this study grew out of efforts to develop a framework to suit the variety of data collected and do justice to the quality of data. The chosen process had to satisfy my need to build, through the evolutionary data collection phases, an interpretation of the whole data and all its constituent parts. It was at this juncture that I realised how I had been using the hermeneutic circle and exactly how it would operate during analysis. At the core of the purpose of the analysis, was the need to seek meaning and make sense of the data, without losing the contextual and individual meanings that were the reality for the participants. Packer and Addison (1989, p141) describe how they developed a reading guide which helped them search for different meanings in their data and the importance of re-reading in order to gain interpretations of different aspects of it. Van Manen (1990), in his explanation of hermeneutic phenomenological reflection, advocates the use of themes in order to explicate notions, focus, 'moments' in a text and researcher insights. Without trying to generalise the experiences that my participants had conveyed, I needed to order the data in some way which demonstrated their journeys through the Diploma of Higher Education in Nursing Studies course. It evolved that the most meaningful way of arranging the data for this study was according to some of the hermeneutic concepts that Heidegger describes associated with 'being', namely 'intentionality', 'thrownness', 'being-in-the-world-with-others', 'temporality' and 'active subject'. These themes were ideal for my purpose, but were not chosen to 'fit' the data. Rather it transpired, that the process students were encountering incorporated these concepts and the data naturally formed within these themes. I believe that I have found the most meaningful way, within a study that claims to use hermeneutic phenomenology, to present the findings emerging from my data.

Formal analysis frameworks

Diekelmann (1990) advocates a team approach to analysing phenomenological data in a quest to 'get the story right' and obtain consensus about interpretation of material. He describes how the analysts achieve textual immersion through reading and re-reading in order to clarify the emerging themes. I considered that this approach was not appropriate as a consensus of opinion was the aim. As a single researcher, the general purpose of the framework was incongruent with my needs and indeed, such a linear process does not satisfy the demands of the hermeneutic circle.

Colaizzi (1978) describes a process which would identify similarities in the data, but does not accommodate the search for uniqueness of experiences. He formulates exhaustive descriptions of the data in order to produce a single representation of the phenomena. For me, this method ignores the importance of individuals' experiences.

Similarly to Colaizzi (1978), Spiegelberg (1960) emphasises general essences rather than the uniqueness of experience. Whilst it has been important to be able to arrange the data in this study thematically, I have also attempted to restore and maintain the importance of each individual's experience.

The aim for Giorgi (1985) is to gain and express psychological insights contained within the data. The perspective is fundamentally psychological, which would have been appropriate for this study, had I used personal construct theory in its pure sense.

However, this study is not concerned with how the constructs were formed by students, but rather why and at what stage of their nurse education they were formed. In addition, I did not have the knowledge or expertise to analyse my data solely from a psychological perspective.

Van Kaam (1966) offers rather a positivistic approach to analysing phenomenological data. Part of the process involves the researcher

60

grouping descriptive expressions within the data which are then agreed upon by expert judges. This implies that there are individuals available who have a monopoly on knowledge associated with the data. This is inappropriate for my study. Van Kaam (1966) also advocates listing percentages and occurrences and testing hypothetical descriptions against a random sample of cases which in my view, would mistreat the data and fail to satisfy the intentions of this study.

It should be acknowledged that clinging rigidly to an existing method in the analysis may force the data to behave in a predictable manner. As a consequence, interpretation can only bring out of the data what the existing method of analysis, based on its points of departure, allows. This may result in a study that is epistemologically conflicting (Haggman-Laitila, 1999).

The final 'formal' phenomenological analysis framework, I considered from the literature, was Reinharz (1983) who describes in broad terms a process of transforming the private experiences of individuals into meaningful written documentation which enables the expression of new understandings (Appendix 8). The process demonstrates an appreciation of uniqueness and the similarities between study participants and identifies the importance of the hermeneutic circle. I found this refreshing after a long, rather demotivating trawl through the qualitative data analysis literature. Selecting Reinharz's framework was not the end of the search for appropriate ways to handle my data. I also had to consider other less formal but just as important options which arose from the nature of the data itself.

Informal analysis frameworks

In order to discover a manageable process, whereby all data collected could be equally treated and explored, I firstly identified the components and actors involved in the research (Figure 3.1). This enabled me to conceptualise the elements and participants and ensure that, whatever processes I chose, all these aspects must be fully integrated. From this figure, I developed three analysis options (Figure 3.2; Figure 3.3; Figure 3.4) which I considered to be available to me for analysing my specific data.

Analysis option 1 (Figure 3.2) demonstrates what I perceive to be a concept-led analysis where the hermeneutic concepts take precedence over the components identified. Keeping these concepts in mind during the analysis, using this option, would ensure that hermeneutics was central to the search for meaning. 'Being-in-the-world', 'Being-in-the-

61

Figure 3.1   Considerations for Hermeneutic Analysis

Students

David
Cathy
Carol
Paula
Sarah
Ben
Clare
Marie

Hermeneutic Concepts

Being-in-the-World
Being-in-the-World-with-Others
Reflection
Active Subject
Intentionality
Situated Freedom
Horizon
Thrownness
Unique Experiences & Essential Themes
Temporality

Methods / Techniques

Questionnaires
Interviews
Repertory Grid Technique
Present Tense Commentary
Reflective Practice Portfolios
Letter Writing
Questionnaires

Me!

Myself as Educationalist
Myself as Practitioner
Myself as Researcher

Figure 3.2   Option 1 – Concept-Led Analysis

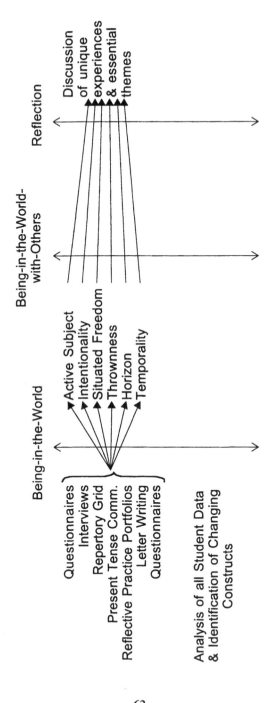

63

Figure 3.3   Option 2 – Student-Led Biographical Analysis

David	=> Q	=> I	=> RGT	=> PTC	=> RPP	=> LW	=> Q	
Cathy	=> Q	=> I	=> RGT	=> PTC	=> RPP	=> LW	=> Q	
Carol	=> Q	=> I	=> RGT	=> PTC	=> RPP	=> LW	=> Q	General
Paula	=> Q	=> I	=> RGT	=> PTC	=> RPP	=> LW	=> Q	Discussion of
Sarah	=> Q	=> I	=> RGT	=> PTC	=> RPP	=> LW	=> Q	Hermeneutic
Ben	=> Q	=> I	=> RGT	=> PTC	=> RPP	=> LW	=> Q	Concepts
Clare	=> Q	=> I	=> RGT	=> PTC	=> RPP	=> LW	=> Q	
Marie	=> Q	=> I	=> RGT	=> PTC	=> RPP	=> LW	=> Q	

Key   Q – Questionnaire   I – Interview   RGT – Repertory Grid Technique
PTC – Present Tense Commentary   RPP – Reflective Practice Portfolios
LW – Letter Writing

Figure 3.4   Option 3 – Methods-Led Analysis

David	David	David	David	David	David	David
Cathy	Cathy	Cathy	Cathy	Cathy	Cathy	Cathy
Carol	Carol	Carol	Carol	Carol	Carol	Carol
Paula	Paula	Paula	Paula	Paula	Paula	Paula
Sarah	Sarah	Sarah	Sarah	Sarah	Sarah	Sarah
Ben	Ben	Ben	Ben	Ben	Ben	Ben
Clare	Clare	Clare	Clare	Clare	Clare	Clare
Marie	Marie	Marie	Marie	Marie	Marie	Marie
→	→	→	→	→	→	→
Q	I	RGT	PTC	RPP	LW	Q

Discussion of Unique Experiences & Essential Themes in Relation to Hermeneutic Concepts world-with-others' and 'reflection' would be integral to the analytical process but not particularly evident in the writing up of findings. I believed that this process would reveal the individual journeys of the students and would be relatively easy to accomplish. The analytical process is neatly sequenced and I like the idea of a general discussion around unique and similar experiences of the students. However, I could anticipate the danger of students' data being presented in isolation because each student data set would be managed separately. There is also the potential that sequential presentation of each student's data might bore the reader.

Analysis option 2 (Figure 3.3) utilises what I call, a student - led biographical analysis, whereby each student's data is analysed and presented, without particular reference to hermeneutic concepts, until the final discussions. Each data collection phase would be analysed for that particular student and themes would be identified vis-a-vis that student and only in relation to that individual's development. It would only be in the final discussions that similarities or uniqueness of experience would be identified. Using this process would enable the developmental nature of the data to be portrayed as well as the changing constructs of each student. There would be an emphasis on unique experience and I felt comfortable with handling the data this way. On the other hand, I felt anxious that the hermeneutic concepts could be lost until the end discussion. Analysing each data set for each student could be repetitive and there is the potential for students to be presented in isolation. This approach would necessitate a separate justification for the use of biography.

The methods - led analysis option 3 (Figure 3.4) would enable me to keep data sets neatly whilst facilitating, comparing and contrasting between each student. I expected that analysis would proceed according to data collection method and this would enable the progressive/evolutionary nature of the data to be exposed. My reflections upon each of the methods would occur naturally, but students' journeys and the experiences contained within the data sets could be disjointed.

I presented these three options to my first and second supervisors who facilitated my exploration of the advantages and disadvantages of each option. After discussion, my only option had been made clear. I had to perform all three - this would lead to a thorough analysis of the data and the comparing, contrasting and in depth exploration of data sets would comprise the hermeneutic circle - the circularity of understanding.

In addition to using Reinharz's framework, as a guide to organise my data and my own informal frameworks to help me process the data, I also used six of Kelly's eleven corollaries [described in Chapter 2] to provide further understanding of the meaning that student's assign to some experiences. Appendix 9 provides a brief explanation of how the six corollaries were interpreted and utilised during analysis of the students' data.

After I had explored the data and a draft of each of the chapters in Part IV had been written, I enrolled the assistance of two of my teaching colleagues to read the drafts. Their remit was to attempt to relate the concepts of intentionality, thrownness, Being-in-the-world-with-others, temporality and active subject to their own experiences as nurses and teachers and also as observers of student nurses' development. I saw this as a means of generating deeper insights and understandings of the students' data. Also, on the basis of colleagues' descriptions, I was able to detect a resonance between students' experiences and theirs (Appendix 10). Van Manen (1990, p100) advocates this process, especially where conversation can, in an informal way, assist the researcher with their interpretations.

Issues of credibility, dependability and transferability

Many authors address standards in qualitative research (Appleton, 1995; Beck, 1994; Burns, 1989; Hinds, 1990; Rose, Beeby and Parker, 1995; Stiles, 1993). These authors concur with Koch (1994) who describes efforts to establish rigour in qualitative research and quotes Guba and Lincoln's (1989) criteria of credibility, dependability and transferability as a scheme to support and authenticate the interpretations of the researcher. Credibility should be integral to any study claiming to use the hermeneutic circle because it is concerned with self-awareness of the researcher and reflexivity. Insights develop as a consequence of using reflection during the research process and revisiting data in the light of that growing awareness. Credibility was also achieved in this study through verification of transcripts and summaries by all participants.

Transferability refers to the degree of 'fittingness' of the data gathered to other similar contexts. I aimed for this by enrolling the assistance of two colleagues who read my interpretations and summaries of students' experiences and by discussing the meaning and application of the interpretations, in terms of their own experiences, with students.

I have also provided a contextual chapter (4), so that other nurse educationalists can compare and contrast their situations with mine and make judgements about similarities and differences in relation to the discussion contained herein.

I aimed for dependability by recording my decisions about the methodology so that the reader has an opportunity to audit the processes. I have endeavoured to rationalise why I have made certain decisions by discussing options throughout the methodology. Sandelowski (1986) argues that it is important for the researcher to describe their horizon in relation to understanding and interpreting data, and I shall be addressing this issue separately in Chapter 5.

Summary

This chapter has provided an overview of the methods and techniques used to collect and analyse data. Where possible, the application of these methods and techniques has been described with particular emphasis on the perceived effects upon the student participants and with regard for the possible consequences for the study in general. I hope to have demonstrated how the methodology adheres to the requirements of hermeneutics and how reflexivity has contributed to my understanding of the students' experiences. In Part III, the contexts in which student nurses experience nursing and nurse education are described to provide a backdrop against which, students' stories are portrayed.

Part III

Contexts and Significant Others

In Part II, I described the processes involved in conducting this study, the underpinning philosophical perspectives and the decisions I made in order that the research demonstrated an allegiance to hermeneutic phenomenology.

In this part it is my intention to introduce the reader to the close context of the research, which I believe has significance for the participants in this study. The 'context' includes qualified nurse practitioners who supervise students during their nursing practice on a day-to-day basis and tutors who teach the students during their time in college.

In addition to these people influencing the students, I have influenced all the processes and people who have participated in this research. Chapter 5 within this Part addresses the issues concerned with my presence as an educationalist, a practitioner and as a neophyte researcher.

4 Perceptions of Tutors and Practitioners

Heidegger (p93) uses the term 'world' to signify the realm, or the domain, in which people live. In the case of my student participants, 'world' refers to the environment and contexts within which they encounter the everydayness of nursing. Heidegger makes explicit the relationship between the phenomenon of 'world' and the sense that individuals assign to experience. Indeed, the importance of context to experience cannot be underestimated using an ontologico-existential approach. Using hermeneutic phenomenology, experience and 'world' should not be separated. It follows therefore, that I have an obligation to the reader to set the scene for this study and to show how the students' 'world' might have influenced their development.

This chapter constitutes summaries of the views of nurse tutors and practitioners concerning nurse education, the selection of student nurses, supervision and the 'new' Project 2000 course. Data to inform this chapter were collected between 1994 and 1995, one to two years after Project 2000 had been introduced to the study area.

This information is included to provide the reader with an insight into the study area, the dynamics occurring between education and clinical practice and the expectations held of students by those responsible for their development into the professional role of the nurse. Focus groups with tutors and interviews with practitioners were seen to be necessary because collectively, these people set the scene for students and are perceived as role models who take part in the students' world on a day-to-day basis. Justification for and processes of conducting focus groups with tutors and interviews with practitioners precedes the discussion.

Focus groups with tutors

All nurse tutors (N=27) working in the college where this study was conducted were invited to attend a focus group to discuss issues related to nurse education, the selection of student nurses, supervision and the 'new' Project 2000 course. Twenty-seven tutors agreed to participate and these individuals were randomly assigned to nine focus groups. The primary aim of the focus groups was to capture the modes of thinking with regard to Project 2000 education and the experiences of tutors involved in facilitation of students' learning. The main areas of exploration included perceptions about how students became nurses and how they were influenced at the beginning of the Course; how and why tutors selected and recruited individuals for the Course and their perceptions of what nursing is and what nurses should be. Because they were randomly assigned to groups, there was an interesting mix of specialisms and professional backgrounds. All tutors provided me with biographical information on a sheet which they signed as a consent to participate.

MaCleod Clark, Maben and Jones (1996) summarised the challenges of using focus group interviews and also provided useful advice on promoting success with the method. These include consideration of group size, access and sampling, the role of the moderator and data analysis issues. However, I chose to ignore advice about group size (Kitzinger, 1994; Macleod Clark et al. 1996 and Morgan, 1988) which generally recommends between four and twelve participants per group. I knew that I would not be able to facilitate discussion with large numbers of tutors. I was aware of the characters of the participants and mindful of keeping abreast of discussions and I also wanted to ensure that each participant had equal talk time. My decision to run nine groups was a wise one on reflection. Each focus group lasted for over an hour and individuals appeared relaxed. I envisaged, with a large group, that the purpose of the discussion might be lost and that general 'chit-chat' might ensue. There is a tendency for us, as nurse tutors, to exploit opportunities of being together to discuss professional issues on a broad front as this rarely happens due to pressure of individual commitments.

Much of the literature associated with conducting focus groups is to be found in Marketing and Business journals. Focus groups have been used in this domain for some considerable time, with the purpose of gaining consensus of opinion regarding products and as think-tanks for new product ideas (Calder, 1977; Kruegar, 1988; Mc Quarrie and McIntyre, 1987; Morgan, 1988). This literature contrasts with more recent nursing research studies which have utilised the method, such as Bailie and Steinberg (1995), Lankshear (1993), Nyamathi and Shuler (1990) and Reed and Roskell (1997). The appeal of the method includes the dynamic nature of the interaction, free exchange of ideas and the cost effectiveness of gaining insight into the opinions of a group of people, as opposed to conducting interviews on an individual basis.

My original intended position within the focus groups with tutors was as an objective interviewer; neither sharing nor disputing the views conveyed by my colleagues. This of course, was unrealistic considering the amount of discussion amongst my colleagues relating to changes within nurse education and the state of flux in the study area in 1994, when these focus groups were conducted. In reality my position was as an empathetic listener who contributed to the material contained in Chapter 4 in response to the membership bestowed upon me by my colleagues in each and every group. This is demonstrated through my understanding of the language and symbols used between tutors and my familiarity with individuals in the groups. Having an awareness of the effects of researcher presence and developing a 'researcher Self' are concepts described by Roberts and McGinty (1995). This concept is explored in Chapter 5, where I have described 'my emerging selves'.

The 'foreknowledge' gained from being an insider was valuable during the processes involved in transcribing the interviews, recognising voices and also in interpretation of the discourse within the transcript text. Webb (1992) refers to dual understanding as "mutual verstehen" where the researcher and the researched are part and parcel of the interpretation which was evident in the focus group discourse.

Many qualitative researchers discuss the position of researcher in the making of data and within the analysis of it (Ashworth, 1986; Greenwood, 1984; Roberts and McGinty, 1995). Not sharing the perspectives, feelings and common sense assumptions of the respondents is thought to lead to misinterpretations and interpretation out of context (Hanson, 1994). Roberts and McGinty (1995) clearly describe the processes involved in being in the data and emphasise the discipline necessary to reflect upon the research, record reflections and critically expose the researcher's development. I hope to have achieved this by offering a precis of my reflections on using this method.

Being reflective is part of reflexivity and has been achieved through examination of my influence in the focus groups; of how my colleagues responded to my presence as being simultaneously an outsider and an insider; through analysis of my thoughts and opinions recorded on my dictaphone and by thoroughly questioning my understanding of each focus group event.

There were occasions where 'dual reflexivity' occurred during the focus groups, where tutors reflected upon experiences and examined their reflections out loud during the focus group process. In response, I reflected and exposed my understanding of experiences to my colleagues. In some ways, this open acknowledgement of my understanding acted as a validating process, whereby my interpretations of others' experiences were exposed.

In addition to being present at the focus groups, I engaged in a dialogue with the verbatim transcripts and, by so doing, became involved all over again. Data analysis of focus group material is given little attention in the literature and I had to decide whether to value each individuals' contribution as unique, or to use the group as the unit of analysis. I opted to use a simple thematic approach whereby common topics were grouped together (Lincoln and Guba, 1985; Miles and Huberman, 1994).

Initially I read the transcripts several times to familiarise myself with their content. This also enabled me to situate myself in the dynamics and processes occurring. I used a code for each individual and numbered each of their sentences throughout the transcript. The core discussion categories for each group were then extracted - a total of 273 categories emerged from the nine groups.

Having revisited the transcripts, I then merged the categories I perceived to be of similar meaning to form 31 themes of significance (Appendix 11). In order to facilitate this 'merging', an overview of all the categories was displayed on the wall. Analysis of this data began in 1995 but I revisited the data, was entertained by it, relived it and provided additional understanding of it in the light of my personal and professional development.

My reflections on this method comprised several pages of what I observed and learned during the process. The following points summarise these reflections;

1. Participants sometimes change or even reverse their original positions during a discussion, having listened to the opinion of others. Is this as a result of enlightenment on their part, or a case of siding with the majority or not wishing to expose a contradictory opinion? I can't imagine that it would be the latter, as there is security in such a small group and I don't believe that any of the tutors would agree with something contrary to their belief.
2. Even with such small groups, I found it difficult sometimes to keep up with the rapid flow of conversation - I certainly did the right thing to use a taperecorder.
3. There are many advantages to sharing a similar frame of reference. Although I have had to ask for some clarification of issues, I understand the terminology and feel comfortable with the overall atmosphere of the groups.
4. It was an effective decision to randomly assign tutors to groups as this has provided interesting discussions from a range of

perspectives. It could also account for some opinions being changed during the conversations.

5. I should have used an orbital microphone, as it has been difficult transcribing the voices of individuals who sat away from the microphones.
6. Starting with a broad question was a good strategy to get people loosened up and communicative.
7. The biographical data sheet helped my understanding of individual perspectives.
8. I feel that my facilitation skills have refined over the nine focus groups and I am now able to approach the method more flexibly.

Interviews with practitioners

Macleod Clark et al (1996, p158) refer to the practitioners in their study as an "important set of stakeholders", implying that those in clinical practice have a vested interest in students. Indeed, the practitioners were seen to carry the major responsibility for imparting clinical skills and preparing students to perform effectively in practice.

Unfortunately, Melia (1987) did not incorporate a practitioner perspective into her study of the occupational socialisation of nurses in the late 1970s. However, there is evidence of practitioner expectations of students in her analysis of students' interview data and these have been useful in providing insights into the changing perspective of the practitioner.

Selecting practitioners for the sample

To access a sample of practitioners for my study, nurse managers of the three local Trusts were contacted in 1995 to request lists of registered nurses. Two of the available Trusts denied access to this information which reduced the available number of registered nurses considerably. The Trust which granted access consists of a general hospital, several community hospitals, mental health units, learning disability units, nursing homes and out-patient facilities. This meant that all placements where students gained experience could be represented through the practitioner sample.

Fourteen hundred nurses were entered into the sampling frame. Fifty were randomly selected and invited to participate in the study. Eight replied to this first request. Because of the poor response, another fifty nurses were randomly selected from the original list. Four replied to this second request. A third trawl brought the number of practitioners, prepared to be interviewed, to fifteen and I considered this adequate to provide contextual data as a backdrop to the students' stories. Whilst this was a disappointing response, I would suggest that the ethos of clinical practice at that time was one of high workload and increasing pressure, accompanied by a diminishing resource allocation and the newly introduced supernumerary status of student nurses. Practitioners may not have had the motivation to participate in a study concerned with nurse education issues, when they were faced with clinical problems of their own.

The practitioner sample comprised fourteen females and one male; twelve RGNs (Registered General Nurses), two RMNs (Registered Mental Nurses) and one RNMH (Registered Nurse, Mental Handicap). They had all been qualified over five years and, with one exception, had supervised students on the Diploma courses for two years. Convenient dates were arranged for one-to-one interviews using a semi-structured guide. At the time of their interview, practitioners completed a biographical data sheet, similar to that for tutors, asking for details about their qualifications and nursing speciality, further study and written consent to use the information.

I outlined the purpose of the study and addressed confidentiality issues with each practitioner prior to commencing the interview. The interview guide consisted of thirteen open-ended questions associated with selection, recruitment, education and supervision of students on pre-registration diploma courses. My questions for the practitioners were similar to those used in the focus groups with tutors, but with an emphasis upon education in clinical practice rather than education in college.

Because of the similarity of questions, I envisaged the potential for contrasting the views of practitioners and tutors. Themes emerging from the practitioner's data can be seen in Appendix 12.

All interviews were conducted at a convenient time and place for the practitioners; these were tape recorded and lasted for approximately an hour. The interviews were transcribed verbatim and transcripts were returned to the practitioners for verification. They were then returned to me, confirming accuracy and without censoring.

My position in these interviews was very different from the way I conducted myself in the focus groups. I recorded very little on my dictaphone as part of my reflective journal during this data collection phase and remember the interviews became rather a chore after the first five. This stemmed from a certain predictability in what practitioners had to say about the 'new' system of nurse education and I found this very frustrating and depressing.

I often felt tempted to enlighten practitioners with my perceptions regarding the advantages of supernumerary status and the application of theory to practice. I was also very conscious of taking their valuable time and this was confirmed by a couple of comments, alluding to busy time schedules and the impending responsibilities of the ward or department. I was however, welcomed by those with whom I had come into contact whilst they had undertaken courses in the college. Despite being randomly selected, out of the fifteen practitioners interviewed, seven were known to me.

It is evident in the interview data that I was not fully accepted as 'one of them' despite my thirteen years of clinical experience. Unlike the focus groups, where I was absorbed into the homogeneity of the groups, I was seen as an interviewer asking questions and expecting answers. I could only try to redress the balance by letting them speak freely, without judgement [although I have not convinced myself that I achieved this] and listening with interest. My presence in the interaction with practitioners manifested as a seeking, probing voice trying to make sense of what they were telling me, whereas my responses in the focus groups were characterised by empathic and confirmatory mutterings. This awareness and subsequent understanding of my position in relation to the data has come about through reflection and a consciousness of the distance developing between my own nursing practice and my current role in education.

Tutors giving support to students

Focus group discussions with tutors centred around two main aspects of support for students; academic support and pastoral care. Tutors agreed that the younger students had more of a problem than their mature counterparts with basic literacy skills, despite having GCSE English Language. Mature students were perceived to have potential to perform at the academic level required, although needing help with academic style. Considerable time was spent coaching 'weak' students in an attempt to improve standards and this was seen to be some kind of rescue fantasy, whereby tutors needed to care for students, which they believed might have occurred as a legacy from the caring role of the nurse. At the time of this study, there was no pre-course study skills module which meant that tutors became responsible for remedial work with students. This role occupied much of their time when they considered they should be offering more advanced academic support. Tutors believed that this type of over-protective behaviour did not occur in mainstream higher education.

There was an acknowledgement that generally students required more support with academic work at the beginning of the Course and less as time went on when they became familiar with the demands of the assignments.

Many students were seen as having insecurities regarding the interpretation and analysis of literature and there seemed to be a fine line between tutors advising the student about aspects of their work and giving so much support that it ended up as a joint effort between the academic tutor and the student. FG15 commented;

They would love me to dictate to them, to think for them and to read for them.

(FG15)

Academic support of students was considered to be a response dependent upon the academic ability of students. Tutors believed that 'A' levels were by no means a guarantee that students would be successful on the Course or achieve the academic requirements at diploma level. Candidates whose selection was based upon five GCSEs, were deemed to lack 'expression' and the ability to construct sentences.

The dilemma of selecting potential students on academic criteria or using a wider entry gate continually arose during the focus groups. Discussions revolved around the notion that any individual should be given the opportunity to prove themselves and become a nurse and the need for individuals to have refined academic skills on commencement of the Course. Some tutors believed that students needed to learn how to 'jump through the hoops', 'play the game' and learn how to satisfy assignment guidelines using the academic support system. There was recognition that candidates needed to demonstrate potential to function at the required level,

otherwise it's a quantum leap from the minimum five GCSEs to diploma level.

(FG18)

There was a perception that tutors had become besotted with academia since the inception of the Project 2000 curriculum and one commented that this might be due to tutors *transferring the demands of the sluice into academia.*

(FG5)

That is, the wideheld belief that nursing is gruelling, punishing work and that the education which gives an individual a licence to practice should be an endurance test.

Academic support was inconsistently defined by tutors, each having their own interpretation of the role and ways of conducting the tutor/student relationship. Tutors acknowledged that students must find it difficult if they receive conflicting advice from different tutors on the same assignment.

In contrast to the intense academic support role, the pastoral role emerged but was considered by some tutors not to be part of their remit;

I spent time sitting outside college with her having a smoke and giving quite deep counselling, which is not what I'm supposed to do really.

(FG 2)

Many students needed five minutes with their tutor just to 'let go' and talk themselves through a situation in practice or if they had been experiencing problems with an assignment. Tutors agreed that often, students just needed time and space and the reassurance that they were doing fine.

Several tutors referred to 'caring' for their students. Although Severinsson's (1996) study was concerned with supervision in clinical practice rather than in the academic environment, the claims that individuals offering support to students should be sensitive to the needs and demands of the students and in particular, show attitudes of "love, respect, hope and confidentiality" (p195) appear to be borne out by the tutors' comments.

FG17 reflected on how the Project 2000 curriculum had demanded a change in the tutor role regarding academic support for students;

A lot of the personal bit has gone. It was not just working as a tutor, but it was the caring bit. In some respects that has gone. Students are quite distant; we don't get to know them. We don't know all their names after three years. Some of the niceties have gone. I think if you're expecting them to be carers, then we have to be caring. I would expect a nurse on the ward to know the names of the patients in her care, but I don't know the names of the students and I equate the two.

(FG17)

Although the pastoral aspect of supervision was recognised and debated, tutors were aware that this attitude to students may well have made them dependent on tutors in the past. The fact that times had changed with tutors no longer 'looking after' students was seen as possibly having an effect on those considering nursing as a career option:

I think a lot more people go [ie leave] *because we don't operate that role. The systems are different because they are all to do with the students having rights and making sure we don't end up in a court of law. But in those days it was more to do with caring and the teaching role, rather than the academic aspect of the teaching role.*

(FG20)

The complex social lives of students were portrayed in the focus group discussions with tutors. They talked about students being homeless and not having enough money, about the effects upon students of having an abortion and difficulties with relationships. They also talked about difficult clinical problems that students brought to the attention of their tutors in the hope that they could resolve them. The involvement of the academic tutor in giving pastoral support in situations such as these, often left the tutor in a difficult predicament, trying to resolve several problems associated with the work and social environment of the student. Giving support to students was seen by tutors to be draining, often repetitive but usually effective in assisting students to recognise their own personal and academic potential.

Practitioners supervising students

The importance of the student-supervisor relationship has been the focus of literature regarding support and the development of skills in clinical practice (Bodley, 1991; Booth, 1992; Flagler, Loper-Pavers and Spitzer, 1988; Ravey, 1992; Twinn, 1992).

During the one-to-one interviews, practitioners described their supervisory role on a continuum from simply a teacher to a more complex amalgamation of counsellor, advocate, defender, mother and guru. None of the practitioners referred directly to their responsibility to students in demonstrating good standards of care, although recognition of their responsibility to act as role models to students formed the basis of the supervisory role. They perceived themselves to be role models for leadership and management skills and to have a responsibility for imparting clinical knowledge. Practitioner 4 admitted knowing little about the Course, but showed insight into the needs of students. Making sure that students received a really good experience assumed priority in her supervisory role. She used the term *comfort* to describe how she intended to provide a secure environment in which students could learn, which she spoke of as *mothering them a bit*. This nurturing aspect of practitioner 4's perception of the supervisory role is balanced by her expectations of students to develop skills and clinical expertise. This type of caring for students was seen to promote 'belongingness' in the ward environment. Practitioner 6 had a similar caring approach to supervision and viewed students as colleagues who negotiated their learning outcomes with qualified staff. She stated *they are one of us*, implying that students are treated as part of the team, from the outset of the placement. This concurs with the findings of Wilson-Barnett, Butterworth, White, Twinn, Davies and Riley (1995) who identified that being included as part of the team and being able to make a contribution were significant influences on whether students felt supported. However, this inclusion of students into the working environment draws attention to the possibility of their losing supernumerary positions. Tutors also highlighted the danger of students being 'thrust' into difficult situations, where they are expected to cope, with inadequate preparation.

The recognition that students should be treated as equals with needs shows respect for them despite the obvious distance in experience and expertise. Closing this gap, through mutual respect, contrasts to the traditional style of nurse education where the student was most definitely subservient to the qualified staff and often felt in awe of them. Consistency, genuineness and respect were identified by Project 2000 students in Cahill's (1996) study as important features of the supervisory relationship with students whereas a clearly defined supervisory role was not particularly important. However, practitioners in my study commented that diploma students often became over-familiar with them as their supervisors and found it difficult to achieve a balance between treating them as superiors or close friends. Practitioner 4 recalled how she was *scared shitless* by qualified staff when she was a student and contrasted this with the attitudes of current diploma students.

Directing students to alternative sources of information was also seen as the supervisor's role in addition to an appreciation of the need to satisfy competencies. Students were often perceived as being selfish and not understanding the needs of those within the placement area. This implies that students arrive at their placements with their own agendas

81

to fulfil, rather than acknowledging that staff and patients within the placement have needs.

Interestingly, supervisors of mental health and learning disability students were more concerned with orientating them to the specialism rather than encouraging immersion as soon as they arrived. This activity by supervisors focuses upon the need for students to appreciate how the areas function on a day-to-day basis; this was seen to be important where patients and clients treat the placement area as their home, or where they stay for long periods of time and this results in the least disruption to the lives of the residents. Practitioners recognised that one of the problems that beset diploma students in practice was the apparent resistance from qualified staff. They recalled incidences where students had been overwhelmed by the *it wasn't like that in my day* syndrome (P14). Many practitioners appreciated that diploma students were *coming at it from a different angle* (P14), but that clinical staff failed to appreciate the change in expectation. Practitioners thought that students in practice feared retribution in their dealings with clinical staff and agreed that this was unfortunate and undesirable.

The supernumerary role caused some conflict in practice, particularly where supervisors took it literally to mean that students could only observe. This led to students themselves being unsure of what they were and were not allowed to do.

The expectation by qualified staff that diploma students would perform equally well in practice as traditional students was thought to present an added pressure for students. Practitioners acknowledged that there appeared to be a general concern for the apparent lack of practical skills demonstrated by diploma students. However, there was recognition that clinical skills could be learned very quickly if the rationale and knowledge associated with the skill had been learned. Practitioners believed that the range and quantity of clinical skills a student is able to achieve often depends upon their personality. It was thought that if the student was outgoing, then they would be more likely to ask and then insist on practising skills under supervision. These students were also seen to be better at organising learning opportunities, thus increasing their exposure to a variety of clinical settings and procedures. In turn, this increased the student's confidence in being able to contribute to the team. Macleod Clark et al. (1996, p146) identify the initial skills deficit but also describe many differences between traditional and diploma students in a positive light. Interestingly, practitioners in my study viewed diploma students as being more 'individual' than their traditional counterparts. The preconception that diploma students would be less able in practice was often dispelled and practitioners were surprised.

I was sceptical at first - I thought in their third year they were going to be absolutely hopeless. But the ones we've had that are on rostered service have been equally as good as the traditional students - which I found a surprise.

(P9)

Practitioners were aware of the common anxiety of diploma students about being able to function at the same level as their predecessors. On the whole, practitioners thought that supernumerary status was really important in giving students a chance to learn the ways of practice without being absorbed into the routine of the area. Being available for students and supporting them was seen also to reduce students' anxiety.

It was evident that those who found supervising diploma students stimulating made efforts to keep abreast with developments and despite finding the role demanding and wearing, enjoyed supervising and teaching very much.

Previous nursing experience

Tutors and practitioners agreed that previous nursing experience might be helpful in preparing students to interact with patients/clients and would enable students to feel *useful* because they could *find things to do* (P13) which in turn, might help them to feel valued. P11 believed that previous experience was very important because it prevented culture shock, as these students already had an understanding of the working ethos. It was believed that students with some previous nursing experience could recognise patients' needs more readily and that any experience dealing with people would be to the advantage of the student. However, previous experience was not always recognised as being positive; practitioners considered that some students with prior experience continued to function at nursing auxiliary level and brought bad habits with them. They found it difficult to re-learn skills which disrupted their existing practices. Particular nursing experiences were seen to be detrimental to professional development. For example, many nursing homes used ritualistic practices: P2 commented;

Some people may have had experience in a dreadful place and the practice could have been terrible, so they come away with this totally wrong impression of what nursing's all about. You hear stories about nursing homes and the practice isn't the standard you would want here. That does concern me and if someone said "I'm waiting to do my training but I'm working in a nursing home", perhaps I would be tempted to say "don't", or "I would rather you came in fresh to nursing.

(P2)

In addition, experience in a nursing home or in a community setting, was not seen by practitioners as being 'clinical' experience.

Student nurse - nursing student

Tutors talked about the differences in students' socialisation into nursing and into the Course. They perceived students embarking on the Course with the expectation of becoming a nurse, but becoming a student in a higher education institution instead. Some referred to the confusion associated with dual citizenship as 'cognitive dissonance'. Tutors expected students to behave in a responsible manner from day one and believed that this conflicts with the general student culture which appears to permit students some freedom and leisure time which causes nursing students some difficulty in knowing where they fit in. FG9 had observed;

Some of them develop what could be considered to be the ordinary behaviour of students, in that they just turn up when they want to. In nurse education this is inappropriate behaviour.

(FG9)

Within the focus groups, tutors stated that students were given a strong message that theory was most important and took precedence over clinical practice. This was thought to have occurred because of the presence of the Student Union and other symbols of mainstream education which the old 'schools of nursing' did not have.

Tutors discussed the ability of students to 'act right academically' which I interpret as meaning that they can self-direct their study, know when to seek advice and guidance and produce work of an acceptable standard. However, the student nurse role, with the nurse role being most predominant, was evident to tutors who had observed students taking on the culture of clinical practice. They had noticed how students adopt a *burn out* (FG18) approach as a result of the perceived powerlessness experienced by practitioners in relation to short staffing, insufficient resources and underfunding.

Understanding the balance of theory and practice on the Course presented some anxiety for the practitioners in this study which seems to have been transmitted to students in their placements. Some practitioners found it difficult to grasp the fundamental concepts of the Course and felt that it was undesirable for students to have time out from clinical practice to study. P2 commented that it *wasn't the 'fault' of the students that they have to have study time*, implying that this might be detrimental to the ongoing development of their clinical skills.

Practitioners sensed that students often found the theoretical aspect of the Course difficult and practitioners generally conveyed amazement at the amount of time students spent in the library and writing assignments. It could be that such perceptions of the Course extend the distance between supervisor and student. However, there was evidence to suggest that practitioners had concern for the students and demonstrated an awareness of the financial problems which many of them had;

A lot of the students work outside of the Course and then they struggle to get their assignments in. We've had girls who don't eat because they don't have any money.

(P13)

Practitioners showed an awareness of the apparent disparity between study related to college assignments and study related to clinical practice for students during their placements. This was manifest in their references to learning about 'the ologies' in college and actually 'nursing' during placements. The majority of practitioners showed an appreciation of the dual role of students they were supervising. One had given students time away from their placement in order to complete an assignment.

In the seventies and eighties learning and working meant that students were governed by service and they found ways of coping with the apparent incongruencies between theory and practice. In Melia's (1987) study, the two roles were segregated because students attended blocks of study in the college of nursing, which enabled them to de-role from one context and take on another set of rules in the other. Students undertaking the Diploma course however, experienced theory and practice running alongside each other with the intention of promoting an association between the two. Short placements interspersed with time in college were seen to be the most appropriate way of encouraging students, now 'owned' by education, to apply what had been learned in college to their clinical practice. The differences then, could be seen as external incongruencies in traditional courses and internal incongruencies in the Diploma course.

'Being a student' and 'being a nurse' in my study, was realised as a different set of incongruencies - fuelled by demands from education and practice, but more to do with the actual role of the student nurse.

Students developing their identity

Tutors discussed the influence of the media on whether people gained an accurate insight into the role of the nurse and healthcare systems. They acknowledged that the media sets out to provide an interesting half-hour drama and not necessarily the realities of the job. Discussions pertaining to perceptions of nursing revolved around the issue of various images portrayed by the media and just how believeable programmes like 'Casualty' really were. Generally they believed that on commencement of the Course students had a traditional image of the nurse in an institutional setting and comments were made about the rarity of seeing nurses in the community or a residential home setting. They perceived that there was a certain amount of disillusionment in students arising from the expectation that they would give 'hands on' care from the outset.

Role models were identified as having some responsibility for students gaining an identity in practice, although this was not the focus of the discussion. Tutors were more concerned with what students were learning rather than how or taught by whom. Again there was seen to be a dissonance between role models in nursing and in academia and a perception that clinical staff were slow to advance academically.

The work of the nurse was seen to affect people's everyday lifestyles and the meaning they assign to health and illness. Recognition that people are greatly influenced by preconceived ideas enabled tutors to make allowances for adjustments during the early stages of the Course. Making a judgement at selection, about whether an individual has an accurate perception of nursing, was deemed to be impossible, despite efforts to do so. Potential students were required to demonstrate insight and understanding about the nurse role and what they would be expecting to do during the Course. FG3 commented that despite attendance at college open days, many still had inappropriate expectations of what the Course would entail.

They come with the expectation of giving hands-on care immediately and are not always clear about the expectations in terms of commitment to their academic work and placements. If a rosy picture is painted, then they get culture shock and that is a sure way of demotivating people and causing them to fall by the wayside.

(FG3)

Part of gaining an identity is to wear the dresscode of that group of people. The media do a good job in making sure that the traditional image of the nurse is kept alive. Tutors believed that as soon as students put their uniform on and go into clinical areas, they take on the role. This was seen as undesirable for mental health and learning disabilities students, who were rarely required to wear their uniform in practice areas. FG14 suggested that early socialisation occurs when students are sent for their uniform fitting at the beginning of the Course which perpetuates the idea that they will be wearing uniform all the time. Practitioners and tutors recognised that students were unlikely to have to don their uniforms during the Common Foundation Programme because of the types of placements they would be attending. Role models in mental health and learning disabilities nursing were perceived to be more liberal in their thinking and less concerned with symbols and status. Yet, by the same token, mental health students particularly were seen to have their own dress code [though not a uniform] and by so doing, to have created their own symbols and status.

Tutors made an inextricable link between 'belonging' and 'identity' and perceived clinical staff as having a huge influence on whether students acquired the identity of the nurse. Students were seen to need to gain their identity as a nurse in clinical practice, and in a desperate attempt to achieve this, they seemed prepared to do anything to please their qualified counterparts. This meant that they could be coerced into doing practical tasks, if it resulted in them feeling that they belonged to the team. To be accepted, the behaviours and practices of that group of people are adopted. So, in order to gain an identity, students were often thrown in at the deep end, struggled, and then felt that by making a contribution to the team, they belonged.

Interestingly, tutors also referred to students belonging to the hospital on the same site as the college in this study. A link between the college and the hospital was seen by some to assist with students belonging to nursing. However, this attitude was found to be particularly irksome to the mental health and learning disability tutors, who reminded others that nursing did not only take place in the institutions.

'Belonging' was also seen to occur when students worked the same shifts as their supervisors so that they could work alongside them and be part of the care team. This was seen to give students the opportunity to learn the *work discipline* (FG12) and the responsibility to turn up for shifts. Promoting this sense of responsibility was seen to assist with students' state of belonging. Tutors identified several of the symbols of recognition and believed that generally, students liked to be identified as student nurses.

Practitioners believed that students felt more settled if qualified staff were 'seen to be doing the work' as opposed to being in the office or at meetings. The practitioners in this study recognised that some of their qualified colleagues did not want students around, were not interested in them and had little knowledge about the Course. They felt that 'wanting students' influenced whether students felt they belonged.

Being confident and familiar with routines was seen to be the crux of whether students felt they were becoming part of the team. P3 highlighted the important influence that nursing auxiliaries had on students. This influence was perceived to be so strong that it could determine whether students settled in and enjoyed a placement, or indeed, whether they stayed in nursing.

Perceived qualities of an ideal nurse

Discussions in the focus groups with tutors relating to the 'ideal' nurse characteristics were valuable as they enabled me to draw some inferences about the types of people and their attributes which were deemed desirable by tutors. I knew that not all tutors were involved in selection and wanted to discover whether assessment at selection was consistent and if indeed there was thought to be a desired personality especially suited to nursing.

These discussions also identified the 'product' as defined by the tutors. To some extent, this background information is useful in providing a context for Chapter 10, where students demonstrate thought processes, problem solving and the development required to be an 'active subject' rather than a passive recipient of orders in clinical practice.

The characteristics identified in the focus groups, constitute three transcribed pages of attributes which I found quite overwhelming. If selection is based upon such a rigorous list of traits, it would be amazing if any individual were selected at all. The characteristics describe a superhuman being capable of demonstrating personal integrity and professional excellence. For ease of portrayal of the desired 'product', I have chosen a montage of quotations from the tutors;

A nurse must be flexible in a number of ways and receptive to the needs of clients and the needs of the organisation. They need to be team players and they have to fit into the ward. They should be able to compromise and be a caring person with a sense of humour. A nurse has to be intelligent, professional and honest, but at the same time, they must be pleasant, trustworthy and willing to listen. They should have effective communication skills and be able to organise care, take responsibility and be reflective in their practice. They should have the ability to overcome and recognise limits of resources, so they need to be resourceful and share a camaraderie with their colleagues. They should be able to justify the care they give and demonstrate an air of calmness and accept everybody as individuals. They should be thoughtful about individuals and not just accept current practice for what it is. A nurse should be assertive and know when to go forwards and when to take a step backwards and know their limitations - and limitations of others, but not to condemn them, but to help them as well. We need visionaries and thinkers and commitment is absolutely essential. A nurse should be friendly and approachable, enthusiastic and motivated. They should have common sense and be considerate, not only in their professional role. They should have creative spontaneity and be open minded and questioning. They should have empathy and remember where they came from, particularly in relation to students. They should be able to argue from a knowledge base and have self esteem. They need to have time and optimism and be 'together' as a person themselves. They should be someone who can act as your anchor and who has a genuine interest and concern for the patient. They should have poise and confidence and patients should feel reassured by their presence. They need to have a human element so that they understand that there are times when rules can be broken for the benefit of the patient. In addition, it's important that they have a life outside the occupational role.

Of course, it is questionable whether the potential to develop all of these attributes is possible. In Macleod Clark et al.'s (1996) study, managers within the nursing service side acknowledged that expectations of newly qualified nurses had always been too high and that it was unlikely that the new diplomate nurses would come out 'perfectly formed'. In the same study, issues concerning post-basic education were raised and teachers, nurse managers and practitioners agreed that Project 2000 students, in much the same way as traditional students, only really start to learn particular skills when placed in a particular clinical environment. I have been unable to identify any other similar expectations for selection of students in the socialisation literature.

A distinction should be made between personal qualities and learned behaviours and skills. This fantasy nurse is created through an amalgamation of traits which individual tutors have encountered during their careers in nursing, but it leads me to question whether there is any other professional group with such high expectations of its members.

FG18 provided a more realistic approach to selecting potential nurses;

I wouldn't look for one paradigm case. You want people with varying qualities. You've got to look at individuals.

(FG18)

The most frequently quoted attribute of the qualified nurse was communication skills. These skills were perceived to be at the core of the nurse's role with patients/clients, colleagues, students and relatives. Communication was seen as a way of 'dealing with people' and included the skills of assessment, diagnosis and teaching, and being aware of the needs of others through conversation and relating to people. Listening to staff and patients was seen to be especially important and having the ability to communicate ideas between staff members was perceived to be one of the key functions of the qualified nurse as leader of a team. Part of listening to others was the opening up of Self to new ideas from colleagues.

Knowledge, in particular to answer students *questions, questions, questions* (P2) was also perceived to be fundamental to functioning effectively as a qualified nurse.

The practitioners also valued motivation as a driving force in the qualified nurse and how this could help sustain them in practice and in facing challenges. In stark contrast, practitioners chose to describe the desired disposition of nurses in three simple words – 'Compassionate', 'kind' and 'caring'.

It can be seen that the expectations of practitioners were conceivably more realistic than those of the tutors. Perhaps practitioners focused on core attributes of the nurse role, rather than idealistic traits as identified by the tutors. These themes emerged from both tutors and practitioners and have been presented here to provide a context against which students' experiences can be interpreted. It is appropriate to add some diary comments I made after an interview with practitioner 7. I found this interview particularly difficult to conduct. The practitioner came with her own agenda which comprised an onslaught on the Diploma course and the students.

The keenness of most practitioners to talk with me and their apparent desire to enhance the experience of students contrasted starkly with practitioner 7. The recording on my dictaphone transcribes as follows;

After the interview with P7, I realised that my experience as a practitioner never emerged during the interaction. In hindsight, this may have occurred as a subconscious effort not to associate myself as a practitioner with her as a practitioner! I really didn't want to be associated with this person in a professional context. I became frustrated and angry and defended the current nurse education system. Despite my initial introduction on the 'phone and subsequent explanations at the beginning of the interview, P7 has no idea of who I am or what the intentions for the research are.

On reflection, I can see that the interview may have provided an opportunity for P7 to vent her concerns about the Course and how it is falling short of her expectations ... Her comment *"do you know they don't do anatomy and physiology anymore"* sent me into a spin, trying to understand where she could have gained this sort of misinformation ...

She talked of the *"new-fangled"* ways of learning and how it did an injustice to nursing ... Her misunderstanding of the Course and how it was designed was evident in many ways - particularly through comments such as *"do you know a lot of them have college places?"* ... This apparent ignorance of the Course being delivered in a college environment and the emphasis on the importance of theory to support practice was evident throughout the interview ... Perhaps her comment that she made after I had switched off the tape worried me the most and I considered the effects of such an attitude on students and the patients/clients. She leant forward and lowered her voice *"Do you know they take men and blacks on these Project 2000 courses?"* I was so shocked by her comment that I found it necessary to spend some time after the interview talking through some of the issues surrounding Project 2000 education and then de-roling from the interview. Because of what I had learned during the interview about P7, I saw fit to inform the relevant link lecturer for the area, suggesting that the placement should be re-audited and withdrew into my researcher role.

It is unfortunate that this chapter ends with negative comments from P7, but I thought it necessary to include her contributions as they may represent other practitioners with the same view. However, they do not represent the majority of practitioners I interviewed in this study.

Summary

The focus group interviews with tutors and one-to-one interactions with practitioners will serve the purpose of providing a backdrop for the students' stories and have direct relevance to them. The perceptions of tutors and practitioners regarding the advantages and disadvantages of previous nursing experience and the existing difficulties for students regarding their identity have also been exposed. Tutors identified academic support as their central role with Project 2000 students and acknowledged that individuals required different levels of support and guidance. The pastoral role of tutors also emerged.

Practitioners also identified their supervisory role as being fundamental to student nurse development, but they too recognised that efforts should be made by supervisors to ensure that students 'belong' to the clinical environment, thus providing students with some 'comfort'.

The next chapter is concerned with my 'emerging Selves' during the processes of this research and how these have been influential throughout the various stages of the study.

5 My Emerging Selves

Just as the diamond is multi-faced, so is the self multi-dimensional.
(Swanson and Delia, 1976, p19)

Although I do not want to be seen as an 'emotional exhibitionist', a term coined by Ellis and Flaherty (1992) to describe the 'unpacking in public' of the researcher's responses to the experience of conducting research, I do want to expose my frame of reference. By so doing, I hope to reduce the distance between the reader and my account here. Some believe that presenting qualitative research challenges claims to a singular, correct style for conducting research (Richardson, 1990) and that authors should not be embarrassed by their own subjectivity because their personal stories serve as a reminder that emotions and experiences are not the exclusive property of research participants. It appears that researchers often feel for their participants and their research and yet they are able to track back and forth between an "insider's passionate perspective and an outsider's dispassionate one" (van Maanen, 1988, p77). This results in fluctuating levels of absorption, detachment and confusion in the management of their multiple Selves and roles.

This chapter is concerned with the ways in which I influenced this study - I have been able to identify 'Myself as Educationalist', 'Myself as Practitioner' and 'Myself as Researcher' throughout the research process and it is inevitable that, given my interest in nursing and education, these multiple Selves emerge during the reflexive nature of the research. My aim is to examine my professional 'Selves' and when and how they manifested and operated. Integral to this chapter is a brief acknowledgement of the importance of reflexivity within the hermeneutic circle and the significance of horizon, fore-understanding, historicity and co-constitution of meaning; these hermeneutic concepts are used in this chapter to describe aspects of my involvement with others.

But first of all I consider it important to declare my 'existing Selves', that is, my historicity prior to embarking upon this research. These existing Selves influenced the way I viewed the research and interpreted the material gathered. I have chosen to do this with simple prose, through which a very brief insight into my biography is provided:

I loathed school,
they tried to teach me about politics and equations.
But even though I was good at hockey,
they said I wouldn't amount to much!

I lived in nurses' homes for eight years -
I enjoyed the companionship and support of my peers.
I moved from place to place, as most nurses do
to gain experience.

I was a midwife in SCBU,
and a sister in medical, surgical and orthopaedic environments.
I recognise my need to be needed,
at school I was seen to motivate under-achievers.

I rowed for the City of Oxford,
Oarswoman of the Year 1987!
The relaxing sound of blades in riggers
provided a balance to hectic hospital life.

I come from a family where 'study' is alien
and so they think I'm mad and sad (in that order!).
But I choose to live my life this way,
enjoying the challenges.

I'm a team player, a social animal!
Some say I'm mischievous and a risk-taker -
I never miss an opportunity,
if the experience will create a memory.

I enjoy high speed -
cars, motorcycles and karts.
"You're like a whirlwind" my colleagues have said,
but also "caring" and "pragmatic".

I think a sense of humour is my greatest asset,
but I can be serious!
I like order, consideration and loyalty,
I hate superficiality.

I was lucky to find nursing,
it has enabled me to realise my potential.

I have had privileged encounters
with many people I hardly knew.

I'm sensitive and fragile,
confident and robust.
I'm touched by concern
and angered by others' expectations.

It was mentioned at primary school
that I should be a teacher;
but I only learned how to learn
when I started nursing.

And now it's a pleasure
to learn and teach
and teach and learn.
I care about the students who care for the patients.

Revealing professional Selves

Meaning in context is thought to be directly related to Self (Benner and Wrubel, 1989; Holden, 1991, (2)) and inextricably subjective (Anderson, Hughes and Sharrock, 1988) so that objectivity as defined by the positivist tradition is perhaps never possible and indeed undesirable in hermeneutic enquiry. The hermeneutic circle of interpretation implies that the researcher is utilising some judgement in the uncovering of phenomena and integral to this is subjectivity. The 'hermeneutic circle' is a metaphor chosen by Heidegger to describe the experience of the researcher moving dialectically between the parts of the research and the whole. The idea is that understanding gained is reciprocal and dynamic.

Allen and Jensen (1990) suggest that a hermeneutic approach offers the scope needed to explore human experience. This experience is undoubtedly highly context-specific and essential subjectivity of the consideration of meaning (Taylor, 1993) is a crucial argument for recognising the need for researchers to openly acknowledge their subjective approach to the interpretation of meaning. Indeed, one of the basic tenets of hermeneutics is not to develop a procedure for understanding, but to clarify the conditions in which understanding takes place (Gadamer, 1994) and this can be achieved through reflexivity.

Amongst the self-concept research literature I found reference to 'possible Selves' (Gagnon, 1992; Markus and Nurius, 1986) and the premiss that an individual's repertoire of Selves can be viewed as the cognitive manifestation of "enduring goals, aspirations, motives, fears and threats" (p954). The domain of possible Selves is thought to be influenced by our self-knowledge, which I interpret as 'insight' and representation of our Selves in the past. This is congruent with the emergent Selves discovered within myself during the research process; my experiences as a nurse, my current experience as an educationalist and my evolving Self as researcher. It appears that possible Selves derive from various socio-cultural and historical contexts and can be constructed by an individual's immediate social experiences [perhaps during data collection phases], or by socially determined and constrained situations, such as hospital and university institutions or status.

I have deliberately chosen the term 'emerging Selves' because it reflects the fundamentals of both Heidegger's 'becoming' and Kelly's changing constructs in the wake of experience. I believe that my emerging Selves have been stimulated by various aspects of the research process and that they, in turn, have influenced the interpretations I have made about the data, the participants and the general progress of the study.

It is important to recall the discussion surrounding the concept of bracketing in Chapter 2, as it has ramifications for my emerging Selves and an influence on how I have dealt with my presence in various situations. My argument is that I am unable to achieve bracketing because of my cultural construction of nursing and education. Wrigley (1995) explains the differences between socially constructed and culturally constructed perspectives and, from this, I understand that it may be possible to set aside beliefs and values which have been socially constructed, but that it is impossible to bracket those beliefs and values that are culturally bound and a part of the Self. I am not a person looking from the outside into nursing and nurse education; I am culturally bound to nursing because, as a professional, it is all I have known for 24 years. What I can do, is demonstrate an awareness of how my Selves operate and give them voices in the context and dynamics of the research process. This is similar to Roberts and McGinty (1995) who had the discipline and courage to reflect upon their research as novices, log their reflections and then reveal their growth as qualitative researchers as they actively engaged in watching themselves critically. Several researchers have debated the issue of a subjective approach in qualitative research (Koch, 1996; Lamb and Huttlinger, 1989; Schutz, 1994; Tilley and Chambers, 1996; Wilde, 1992) and generally agree that recording personal development as a neophyte researcher provides a counter argument to those who believe that "researchers lack critical distance in familiar environments" (Ashworth, 1986), "researchers find it increasingly difficult to suspend his or her perceptions" (Hammersley and Atkinson, 1983) and that "researchers stay away from settings in which they have a direct personal and professional stake" (Bogdan and Taylor, 1984). These authors appear to ignore the central premiss of phenomenological philosophy which is that no one is 'value free' and thus it would be virtually impossible to be objective no matter who was conducting the research.

These issues are associated with the doctrine of reflexivity which argues that

> one is free to choose personally relevant aspects of research to draw on and make explicit and to include personal experience and enjoy the wisdom and companionship of the participants.
>
> (Bannister, 1981, p199)

Koch and Harrington (1998) recommend that readers of research examine the text closely for incorporation of voices other than the voice of the lone introspective researcher and that many voices and their influences be recorded. This requires ongoing self-critique and self-appraisal which eventually shapes the research and brings the interest of the researcher to the work.

The emergence of 'myself as educationalist'

'Myself as educationalist' was exposed most noticeably during the focus group interviews with my peers whilst gaining data for Chapter 4. This phase occurred prior to collecting any data from the study participants at a time when I felt inexperienced and insecure in the role of researcher and more comfortable in my role as an educationalist.

Much of the literature on focus groups, especially from the market research field, assumes that participants in the group do not know each other and that the researcher is also unfamiliar to them (McQuarrie and McIntyre, 1987; Mendes de Almeida, 1980). This is in marked contrast to the way they were used in this instance, where the focus groups constituted small groups of individuals who not only knew each other but had also worked together for a considerable time. Nyamathi and Shuler (1990) acknowledge that this can change the group dynamics and recommend that this type of information should be reported when describing the technique.

At the beginning of each of the nine focus groups, I purposely adopted a strategy of brainstorming ideas onto a whiteboard. Instead of formal introductions between people who already knew each other, I believed the time would be better spent identifying key areas for discussion, within the topic areas I had already selected, and of which participants had prior notice. This enabled me to adopt a role in the group that I felt at ease with and enabled the participants to recognise and understand the opening intent of the focus group. The strategy seemed to fulfil my expectation and all participants relaxed very quickly into discursive mode. I also felt that this could be a way of endearing myself to the participants - that I was not situating myself in a role which they found unfamiliar, rather I was seeking information from them as one of their peer group. It also encouraged all group participants to contribute from the outset and had an 'ice breaker' effect.

Some of the most obvious examples of my educational role in the focus groups occurred during conversation with specific reference to educational principles or language.

For example I asked "When you say 'hands on' experience, would it be fair to say experiential?" (FG2, p4) and "You were putting it within a framework for reflection weren't you H?" (FG2, p23).

I also introduced educational terms such as 'androgogy' to summarise statements made by focus group participants and then asked for confirmation that that was what they meant.

Often I would suggest a word to finish a sentence and then seek agreement;

(FG16)   *... It's better than NVQ's and everything else we've got out*
             there where we're not actually able to monitor ...
(Theresa)   ... no control? ...
(FG16)   *No control or anything, at least we need to maintain*
             control.

and regarding desirable qualifications at selection;

(FG7)   *... It would have to be at least an A or a B for English.*
(Theresa)   At GCSE?
(FG7)   *Yeh, GCSE.*

and in relation to references for applicants to nursing;

98

(FG12)	*Sometimes the references are useful and sometimes they are completely inappropriate - it depends on who's written them and the relationship they have with the applicant.*
(Theresa)	... like 'This person is nice and would make a good nurse'?
(FG12)	*Yes - 'ideally suited to nursing', things like that.*
(Theresa)	and 'they won't make it to university but they would be a good nurse'?
(FG12)	*Yes.*

and in discussion about the old 'O' Level system of examination;

(FG5)	*There was no learning in the old 'O' levels, it was just ...*
(Theresa)	Regurgitation?
(FG5)	*Yes, regurgitation.*

In addition to sharing educational language these quotations also demonstrate my understanding of the processes. In focus group 1, I asked a participant "Does that include the open days we give?", after her explanation of strategies for recruitment. I used my knowledge of the processes to seek further information;

"Do you think in view of ..." (FG2, p35) and to confirm that I was receiving their message - "I know exactly what you mean" (FG2, p38).

Sometimes the participants inadvertently drew me into the conversation, especially when it appeared that their answer was not directly related to my questioning. I believe they were not seeking my approval, rather they were treating me as their colleague - they were interested in my opinion.

(FG19)	*The media obviously makes a contribution to their perception of what nursing is.*
(Theresa)	In terms of what?
(FG19)	*Well, Casualty obviously has a major influence and all those images in the newspapers.*
(FG18)	*The things like ER are wonderfully entertaining.*
(Theresa)	I can't bear it.
(FG19)	*It's very slick and the pace is fast.*
(Theresa)	I've never seen so much happening.
(FG19)	*You're dragged into it and it wrings you out.*
(Theresa)	Casualty is more realistic.
(FG19)	*Yes, I think it is too.*
(FG18)	*Maybe that's why it's so frightfully dull.*

(FG19)	*But there's also Cardiac Arrest! which presents a very different image of nursing. Have you seen that?*
(Theresa)	No, I haven't.
(FG18)	*It's very black and gives a ...*
(FG19)	*... negative view of nursing.*
(FG18)	*But people in the profession love it.*
(Theresa)	Do they?
(FG19)	*Absolutely.*
(FG18)	*It's very real in some aspects, but exaggerated.*
(FG19)	*That's right.*
(FG18)	*But very real.*

This type of general 'chat' infiltrates the serious conversation between the participants as if they need to include me in the discussion. Analysis of the focus group data has revealed that I never directly gave an opinion or a stance on a debatable issue.

Sharing horizons

To compose the groups, I used random allocation so that teaching staff were not separated into nursing specialities or teaching teams. There were some interesting mixes of backgrounds, personalities and opinions, but I found it most useful to have knowledge of each individual and their particular foibles and idiosyncrasies. This enabled me to understand their frame of reference and interpret their experiences 'in context'.

Often we shared experiences of our own training days and I concurred with what my colleagues were contributing to discussions. I did not see this as contaminating the data. I was not confirming what they had said was 'right' in any way, simply showing that I understood their horizon and had empathy with their situation. Statements such as "Yes, absolutely", "I would agree", "It is rewarding, yes", "I know what you mean", "Me too!" suggest that I share a certain 'relatedness' to the participants. My familiarity with all participants is evident through continual use of first names during the focus groups and the topics of conversation that initiated discussion, maintained interest and summarised feelings at the end. This familiarity also enabled me to distinguish between potential threatening and non-threatening situations which occasionally arose between participants who had dissimilar opinions. If I detected some antagonism between teachers, I would diffuse the situation by openly accepting each viewpoint and swiftly moving on to the next discussion topic. There was an occasion where two teachers, who often worked together, had a misunderstanding during a discussion about access to nursing courses;

(FG14)   *... we just cream off the people with 'A' levels and it's a total hypocrisy.*

(FG15)   *Oh right!*

(FG14)   *We need to be looking at it representatively in terms of mature students, students from ethnic backgrounds, social class ...*

(FG15)   *It sounds to me as if you're going to go out there with a net, drop the net and bring in everybody and hopefully there will be ethnic people, disabled people, poor people, rich people, intelligent people - is that what you're saying?*

(FG14)   *No. I'm saying that access to nursing is a way of enabling people who may not have achieved. But they have to be able to demonstrate academic ability because look what happens when they get here. I spent hours and hours and hours with someone who just couldn't string a sentence together.*

(FG15)   *But she had 'O' levels!*

(FG14)   *No she didn't. It caused me all this work - then she blamed me!*

(FG15)   *Hang on ...*

(FG14)   *I don't think she ...*

(FG15)   *Hang on ...*

(FG14)   *I don't think she could have ...*

(FG15)   *Hang on ...*

(FG14)   *I thought, why did they select the bugger!?*

(FG15)   *Shut up!*

(FG14)   *I wasn't involved in it so ...*

(FG15)   *I'm confused ...*

This scenario demonstrates my lack of interference during the altercation between participants 14 and 15. I felt confident, knowing both individuals and their favourable working relationship, that there was no threat to either party. In fact the tone of the discussion became that of amusement rather than menace.

I also shared moments of humour as 'myself as educationalist' with my peers during the focus groups;

(Theresa)   If I were to state it on a more personal level, what type of individual would you want caring for you, say if you had

101

major surgery?

(FG18)	*I'd want a good surgeon!*
(FG20)	*I would want to know that the nurse who's caring for me has the same cognitive abilities as a mental health nurse.*
(FG18)	*That low a standard! I'd want a bit better than that, I would want them to have a PhD in epistemology and a knowledge of existentialism!*
(FG20)	*This is true!*
(Theresa)	I hope I can spell all these words when I transcribe this tape.

Toward the end of each focus group, I appeared to rush the last topic for discussion, particularly if the time agreed had elapsed. I was mindful of my colleagues' workloads and tight time schedules. At times I felt that they might be scrutinising my novice researcher traits, challenging me to draw the discussion to a close. However, at no time did I feel unsupported by my colleagues, rather they gave me license to explore the new role of 'myself as researcher'.

This seems to be an appropriate adjunct to introduce the concept of 'fusion of horizons' as defined by Gadamer (1976). An horizon is a perspective, or a way of understanding, which sets the scene for interpretation. We each have many horizons, depending on the influencing stance, and these are considered to be 'temporal'. That is, they develop and change over time. The task in a hermeneutic study, is to show how fusions of horizon occur through depicting expressions in the social context and the way in which the researcher and participants come to share common understandings (Hekman, 1983). From this perspective, understanding takes place against a background of pre-understandings that make our own prejudices, which are then situated against or alongside the text, in order to illuminate it (Walsh, 1996).

Fusion of horizons occurred less spontaneously with the fifteen practitioners I interviewed when gaining an understanding of their perspective for Chapter 4. As 'myself as educationalist' I felt a detachment from the practitioners which I had not experienced during the focus groups. This surprised me, as I held the belief that I was a nurse first and a teacher second. As a result of these interviews, I became aware of my strong attachment to and role within education. During the late stages of data collection my roles changed priority again - teacher first, researcher second and nurse third. As I write up my research I realise that my educationalist and researcher roles are entwined and complementary, but that 'myself as practitioner' will always be the foundation upon which the others depend.

Whilst there is evidence of 'myself as practitioner' in the transcripts, I never had the temptation to be drawn into the conversation. 'Myself as educationalist' is apparent through supporting, encouraging, correcting, educational 'speak' and through offering information during the practitioner's interviews.

(P3)   *Once I decided I wanted to be a nurse, I was studying A levels, I stopped because I thought I wouldn't need them. But now I wish I had because I could go a bit further, which I don't think I can now and get to diploma level which is what they're doing.*
(Theresa)   You don't think you can?
(P3)   *No.*
(Theresa)   Course you can. We can talk about it later.

Practitioner 4 also requested some support;

(P4)   *I haven't got a clue about Project 2000.*
(Theresa)   Right.
(P4)   *I need information, I need someone to come and talk to me about what Project 2000 is and what it means. I know the basics like you do 18 months and then you branch off.*
(Theresa)   Yes, well in fact we can talk about this after the interview. Would that be OK?

As already mentioned in Chapter 4, Practitioner 7 appeared not to connect me with the College at all, despite my explanatory letter prior to the interview. 'Myself as educationalist' became very unnerved by this practitioner's apparent lack of understanding about current nurse education. She continued to talk about how she did not agree with the new Course and how 'useless' the new students were. The transcript shows very few confirmatory utterances from me because I was so amazed and dumbfounded. I listened for some 20 minutes and then 'myself as educationalist' had to defend the new Course;

(P7)   *...I think you do need to have a good knowledge of biology and anatomy and physiology. I can't quite accept it if they drop that after all the years I studied.*
(Theresa)   We haven't! I don't know where you have got that information from.
(P7)   *Oh they say you don't have to do A & P now. They tell me.*
(Theresa)   Well, we can talk about that afterwards.

(P7)   *Perhaps you can enlighten me on why they do these courses?*

(Theresa)   I will, but I'll turn this off first. [Referring to the taperecorder and anticipating a long session explaining the purpose and intentions of the 'new' course].

It is also interesting to note that P7 refers to *they* as the educationalists and yet does not perceive me as a member of that group. I respond by showing some ownership of the Course and including myself as educationalist - "we haven't!".

There were other examples of my educationalist Self, willing to give snippets of information so that the practitioners could continue with their responses.

Practitioner 5 asked;

(P5)   *I think mature students have every right to do the DC test - have they got rid of that?*

(Theresa)   It's on the way out, yes.

Again 'they' does not appear to include me in the group. Several practitioners needed to know more about the entry qualifications so that they could comment on their perceived appropriateness. This may be an indication that the conceptual level of questioning was not always suited to the interviewees' horizon.

My educational 'speak' infiltrated the course of conversation with some of the practitioners in a more subtle way;

(Theresa)   ... That's really brilliant - So that's an outcome that can't be measured but it is certainly noticeable isn't it?

on another occasion;

(Theresa)   I wonder if you have more abstract thinkers in learning disabilities nursing than concrete thinkers?

This was a comment in response to a learning disability practitioner who claimed that most learning disabilities nurses were *gabby, outgoing and extrovert.*

'Myself as educationalist' also assumed a correcting role whereby practitioners who had been misinformed were reinformed;

(P12)   *I was anxious not knowing what level they would be coming out at. They come out (of college) after, what is it, 18 months?*

(Theresa) Not here, they come out after three weeks.

This 'correcting' also occurred when practitioners struggled for educational terminology, such as Practitioner 1, when she called the student assessment documentation 'records' and then looked at me for confirmation and I replied "competency booklets". She also referred to new recruits to nursing being "school leavers" and I counteracted this claim with "only half our students come from sixth form at school or college".

During the interview with Practitioner 14, she talked about not wanting to refer students on their clinical placement assessment. In response to her statement 'myself as educationalist' appears patronising, albeit unintentionally;

(P14)   *It makes you feel such an ogre when you're doing it.*

(Theresa) But we find in college, that clinical staff are very bad at referring or deferring students because they tend to be too kind.

Disparate horizons

These examples of 'myself as educationalist' during encounters with the practitioners demonstrate how my educationalist's horizon operates and manifests itself with a different interest group. This 'Self' also emerged during my many interactions with the student participants. Despite making many attempts to redress the power balance, there were occasions where I took an 'encouraging', 'confirmatory' and 'reassuring' role. However, it could be argued that any researcher, regardless of background, might demonstrate these traits.

In Chapter 3, I attempted to explain how I chose methods and techniques to gather data which addressed the perceived power imbalance between myself as a teacher and the student participants. This perception arose from comments that students have made over the years I have been a teacher and was confirmed to some extent by a student's statement that *tutors are something above* (Ben, one-to-one interview).

I have been conscious of the ramifications of my position within the College and subsequently, the university, and have made efforts to treat students as my equal, as they should be. At the beginning of this study I was a smoker which set me in the advantaged position of sharing idle chat with students during coffee breaks. I felt that the status attributed to 'myself as educationalist' was weakened during these meetings of shared habit and interest. When I gave up smoking, I lost and missed these valuable informative opportunities to mix and gain insight into the social lifeworld of students.

Within the student participant's transcripts, there is evidence of 'myself as educationalist' praising student achievement. This often resulted from them telling me about their assignment grades, appearing to seek approval from me as a teacher or simply because they had performed well, during some of the more complex data collection phases. These congratulatory remarks were not meant as approval, but rather as a 'thankyou' for your efforts. For example; "You're doing this really well", "That's fine", "Good, you've really moved on", "You're grades aren't bad - well done", "You're absolutely right" and "That's great!".

Some of my teacher behaviours occurred naturally, for example during the Present Tense Commentary phase I encouraged students to compare and contrast their positive and negative experiences in order to identify the differences. I also summarised what they had said in previous paragraphs in an effort to clarify and seek verification.

In my composite reflective summaries, written after the Present Tense Commentaries, 'myself as educationalist' is revealed as a maternal self-gratifying persona. I recorded feeling 'proud' that students had developed caring attitudes based on knowledge gained in college and felt that this was a rewarding aspect of teaching. I also made a few judgements about the student's confidence and my perception of their ability to progress and succeed on the Course against criteria I had formulated from characteristics of other successful students I had supervised.

It is difficult to identify the exact point at which our horizons met. I believe that we had many shared understandings particularly in the latter phases of data collection when students felt more relaxed in my presence and a rapport had evolved. There is evidence of shared humour and understanding of the Diploma course and my continual checking to ensure that my interpretations are accurate; "so what you're saying is...", "am I right in thinking ...?", "is that because you just said....?". These examples demonstrate my attempts to reach what Warnke (1987, p169) refers to as "dialogic consensus". Understanding takes place when the horizon of the other intersects or fuses with our own horizon and as a result, changes or extends the range of vision (Walsh, 1996).

> Fusion is the coming together of different vantage points. The process leading to fusion of horizons is more like a posture, or a way of conducting yourself, a willingness to open yourself to the standpoint of another so that you can let their standpoint speak to you, and let it influence you.
>
> (Koch, 1996, p177)

In this study, the fusion of horizons between the student participants and my Selves strengthened at each phase of data collection because my insight into their lifeworlds was more informed at each stage as a result of the previous one. However, I also believe that there is evidence of a non-fusion of horizons in the student data, where I struggled to understand the position held by Carol;

(Theresa) At our last meeting you recognised that you should have done more reading?

(Carol) *I still should.*

(Theresa) ... and you still should? What is it that stops you from doing the reading?

(Carol) *My laziness most of the time.*

(Theresa) What can you do about that Carol? [smiling]

(Carol) *Be more motivated.*

(Theresa) Do you think it's important to have knowledge?

(Carol) *I think it's very important, definitely.*

(Theresa) So is it a personal thing - why aren't you doing it?

(Carol) *It's just laziness.*

(Theresa) And yet you're anxious about writing essays - do you think there's a link here?

(Carol) *It's my lack of motivation.*

(Theresa) What would give you that motivation?

(Carol) *An assurance that I will pass this Course.*

(Theresa) Do you always feel like this?

(Carol) *I'm always like this.*

(Theresa) OK.

'Myself as educationalist' is the predominant role in this encounter, obviously because of my position as senior lecturer and the length of time I have been teaching. Analysis of the instances where this Self has emerged has indicated to me how the role infiltrates most of my interactions and reactions with, and to, various people and situations.

Because of this, efforts to detach from this Self could not be detected in the data and indeed, I believe that to do so would remove the basis of the interpretations contained within this study.

The following section is concerned with a fading, but relevant and significant Self.

The emergence of 'myself as practitioner'

The practitioners had arranged their time so that we had an uninterrupted hour [in theory] and there was only one interview where this privacy was not maintained. I had sent letters to all participating practitioners, informing them of my intention, the aims of the study and possible outcomes and my position in the college.

I felt comfortable in all the clinical environments - even in mental health and learning disability areas which were unfamiliar to me. I was not fazed by aromas, equipment, wandering patients or clients or by members of staff. I felt 'at home'. At the time of conducting these interviews, I had been out of full-time clinical practice for five years, but had maintained a familiarity through a 'link tutor' role. I had developed close relationships with practitioners in my own areas and gained an understanding of the irritations, concerns and satisfactions of nurses at this particular time. They did not appear to be any different from the ones I had found as a nursing sister in 1989. I presumed there would be a relatedness between the practitioners' experiences of supervising students and my own reflections on the activity.

Transcripts of these interviews with practitioners demonstrate a tenuous association between the practitioners and me. I rarely emerged as 'myself as practitioner' and only shared occasional similar experiences. However, I demonstrated an understanding of their responsibility in practice, as with practitioner 4;

(P4)   *Do you mind if I just look out the door?*
(Theresa) Not at all.

Pause and P4 returns

(Theresa) No crises at the moment?

My awareness that an emergency could develop in the space of two minutes demonstrated my empathy with the role.

Practitioner 11 commented that students found working at the

108

weekends, Bank Holidays and Christmas very tiring - 'myself as practitioner' retorted "Welcome to the real world". This type of response is in conflict with 'myself as educationalist' who would argue that students should not be working these shifts unless they had negotiated with their supervisor and there was specific experience to gain. Benoliel (1977) writes of the role conflict which can occur for the nurse researcher in clinical practice and discusses the need for the individual to make a choice between roles. It is quite apparent, in the data, that I remain firmly based in education, with tokenistic connection to the practitioner role. I believe I behave in this way just to share a loose frame of reference with the practitioner participants in order to gain some recognition as being on their 'side'.

Wilde (1992) challenges the conventional rules advocated for researchers undertaking qualitative research (Chenitz and Swanson, 1986). In her research, Wilde acknowledged that she brought with her a number of other roles that she had assimilated during her career. These roles contributed to the 'luggage' that she carried with her "some of these belongings being near the surface and often used, and others being located more deeply but still accessible" (Wilde, 1992, p239). Like Wilde, I have internalised so many aspects of my occupational roles, that they have become 'me'.

'Myself as practitioner' was also remote during the focus group interviews with my peer groups. Although we shared reflections of our 'time' in clinical practice, the emphasis was on educational roles and responsibilities. However, there is always a respect for clinical specialisms in education and each of us was aware of the others' area of perceived expertise. During the focus groups, any reference to nurses in clinical practice was made through the lens of education. They were seen to have characteristics, they were 'good or bad supervisors', 'practitioners had very little time to attend courses', 'they did their best in the current climate'. Educationalists demonstrated an awareness of the practitioner role, but had little empathy with it.

In the early one-to-one interviews with students, it appears that I had a strong need to impress upon students that I had been a nurse. I recorded in my reflections after the interviews, how surprised I was to learn that students did not perceive the tutors to be nurses. In fact I was horrified! This need manifested itself in the question - "how do you view the tutors?". I was angling for students to explore the concept of role modelling and how teachers apply theory to practice in the classroom. 'Myself as practitioner' needed to raise the students' awareness that all tutors were also nurses as I believed it would raise our credibility amongst the student fraternity. It was my perception, at this time, that students had an affinity with nurses in clinical practice to the detriment of education.

The most poignant demonstration of 'myself as practitioner' occurred when the students used the Present Tense Commentary technique to portray clinical experiences to me. I had expected these commentaries to be a time of emotional exposure for the students but had not really anticipated the effect they might have upon me.

In my composite reflective summary of Ben's commentary I wrote;

I share a similar guilt to Ben about leaving people exposed, who are in an especially vulnerable position. As a nursing auxiliary I used to 'toilet' elderly people as if they were on a production line. My lack of compassion now makes me feel disgusted with myself.

(Nov. 95)

Later in the summary I recall 'myself as practitioner';

These stories also remind me of a particular occasion when a patient I had looked after when I was a sister, died. He died from leukaemia and I felt totally helpless. I cried behind the nurses' station where I thought no-one would find me. A student nurse came up to me and said "I would have thought you wouldn't let that sort of thing affect you any more". I felt humiliated.

(Nov. 95)

The stories told during the Present Tense Commentaries transported me back to my own experiences in clinical practice and I remembered the sadness that often accompanied my work as a nurse. Gadamer (1975) contends that understanding involves the application of the text [story] to the situation of the researcher - they must bring the text into an intelligible relationship with their own cultural milieu. This fusion of horizons acknowledges the positions of both the teller and the researcher in relation to a shared frame of reference. I did not force this fusion or mutual understanding; rather it occurred naturally as the students' story unfolded. A fusion of horizons not only occurs between individuals, but as a continuous fusion of the historical horizon with the horizon of the present.

The human connection explained above is referred to as 'co-constitution' (Gadamer, 1975) and is linked to the concept of fusion of horizons. To discover meanings that other individuals ascribe to certain experiences or situations, researchers must not become detached but endeavour to interpret their participant's construction of reality.

110

The emergence of 'myself as researcher'

This reticent Self emerged in the main through behaviours and actions rather than through verbal communication, unlike my other Selves, which could be detected in the transcripts. This Self required much more of a conscious effort to emerge at the outset of this study, but my confidence and development in this role is apparent through my more subconscious attending to research process detail and consideration of issues associated with the role.

In the focus groups with my peers, I suppressed 'myself as researcher' for fear of being isolated from the groups and treated as an outsider. This could have happened if I had not used an ice breaker technique to initiate discussion or if I had become aloof in my interactions with the group participants. In my reflections after the focus groups, I recorded observations associated with the processes involved in conducting the technique. I noticed in the transcript that I had purposely laid tracks for myself through the discussion, in order to make transcribing easier. I was very aware that I might have some difficulty distinguishing voices and often used participant's first names in my efforts to make identification easier. I used this strategy more comprehensively in the RepGrid encounters with student participants when they worked through the grid at their own pace. I left myself signposts during conversations with the students so that transcribing would be easier. For example "This one is about uniform ...", or "are you missing the next one?", "What did you mean by student nurse stigma?"

I also reflected upon my preparations as a researcher - for instance in the focus group interviews I learned that a tape recorder with a microphone at each end was ineffective with five people seated in a circle around it. An orbital microphone would have been more effective in picking up all voices. This made 'myself as researcher' more efficient in preparing the interview environment. However, with practitioners, much of the environment was out of my control, as they chose the venue. During one interview we were interrupted a total of seven times which became very irritating to 'myself as researcher'. On another occasion interviewing a practitioner, 'myself as researcher' interrupted the participant so that I could ask the people who had gathered outside if they would mind keeping the noise down. I was afraid that I would not be able to hear the quiet voice of the participant over the cacophony outside. A group of porters had amassed to spend their breaktime together!

'Myself as researcher' also emerged subtly when I showed care to the student participants in particular. When Clare became upset and started crying about her accommodation problems, I stopped the tape and we went and had a coffee together. At a later stage Cathy asked "can we stop a minute?" and the taperecorder was regulated according to student request.

As 'myself as researcher' I was constantly aware of the effects of the data collection methods and techniques had upon the students. For the most part, I supplied guidelines and examples of how these might be used. At the beginning of each stage I asked the students how they felt using it and any problems or difficulties that they experienced. I was conscious of the time and effort they were willing to invest in my research and wanted to make the interactions useful to them as well as enjoyable.

With reference to the RepGrid;

(Theresa) Do you think this is a good way of collecting information?
(Cathy)   *I do, because it has made me think about it.*
(Theresa) Different to just interviewing you again?
(Cathy)   *Yeh, it made me think about my progression.*

and also the Present Tense Commentary;

(Theresa) *Did you use the reflective framework at all?*
(Carol)   Yeh, definitely, I couldn't have done it without it.

and after using the technique;

(Theresa) How did you find talking in the present tense?
(David)   *I find it quite easy, because while I was doing it I had the situation in my head. I don't think I could have done it any other way.*
(Theresa) OK that's fine - do you want to say anything else about it?
(David)   *I enjoyed it ... it was no trouble at all.*

'Myself as researcher' constantly checked how effective the methods and techniques had been and recorded the student's comments regarding their user-friendliness.

In preparation for the Present Tense Commentary, I had the foresight to arrange a counsellor in case the students were upset or disturbed by their relived accounts. 'Myself as researcher' anticipated that taking on a counselling role and becoming therapeutically involved

112

with the students, could have compromised the student's development and aspects of the study. The dilemma of being over-supportive and dealing with participants' feelings and memories, evoked during an interview situation, is acknowledged by Wilde (1992). She claims that the role of researcher should be kept separate from a clinical role as the function of the research interview is quite different and should not be used for purposes of intervention.

Whilst analysing the Reflective Practice Portfolios, I found it necessary to detach 'myself as educationalist' from 'myself as researcher'. My usual role with the portfolios is as a marker, looking for reflective skills and depth and quality of analysis of experiences and related learning. 'Myself as researcher' was looking for something quite different, particularly in relation to the students becoming autonomous practitioners and myself gaining research material. To ensure that I was satisfying my researcher agenda and not an educationalist one, I kept a list of keywords, identified roles and the aims of the chapter beside me during analysis. Using Reinharz' (1983) hermeneutic analysis framework also prevented me from straying into the role of 'myself as educationalist'.

Summary

In this chapter I have attempted to demonstrate the dynamic processes through the functioning of my various Selves.

The notion of the unitary Self, of a singular, cohesive and essential identity has been deconstructed by feminist authors (Alcoff, 1988; Weedon, 1987). They challenge the idea that individuals have an authentic core or pure essence which is timeless. Rather, their thought traces the constitution of the subject within an historical framework. Explaining the emergence of my perceived Selves within this chapter has enabled me to realise exactly why I am unable to bracket and suspend my fore-understanding. There is consistent and persistent interplay of my Selves in the data and as part of the context shaping my interpretations.

Part III has given the reader some insight into the dynamic nature of the contexts in which student participants in this study have had to operate. The influence of tutors and practitioners upon the development of students into nurses, within a college and clinical environment, has been superficially addressed. However, the perceptions of these key groups of people have been noted and can be used as a starting point in understanding the student nurse's lifeworld. My emerging Selves have also been identified and exposed within the study framework as a whole; as an important part of the methodology and within the context of the students' learning.

Part IV is concerned with the experiences of student participants as they encounter the journey to become nurses. It is structured according to key Heideggerian concepts with each chapter showing concern for an aspect of the student nurses' lifeworld. A characteristic of Part IV is the absence of a staged process of 'becoming', unlike the socialisation literature which generally proposes a defined process with stages through which all individuals pass. The data I collected do not bear testimony to this process.

Part IV

Being and Becoming a Nurse

Having described the contexts which have had an influence upon the participants in the study, and exposed the perceptions of significant others with concern for the professional development of student nurses in Part III, it is now appropriate to introduce the students to the reader. The following chapters within Part IV relate to the hermeneutic concepts of 'intentionality' (Chapter 6), 'thrownness' (Chapter 7), Being-in-the-world-with-others' (Chapter 8), 'temporality' (Chapter 9) and 'active subject' (Chapter 10).

Part IV is concerned with the experiences of the student participants at various times during the Diploma of Higher Education in Nursing Studies course and the meanings they assigned to those experiences. The chapters draw on all the material gathered from participants over a three year period and vary in length according to the nature of the phenomena. Chapter 8, for instance, is lengthy because it is sub-divided into four sections to accommodate a large amount of data. Chapter 10 however, is short in comparison because it deals with a more advanced aspect of clinical nursing practice which was less common in the data.

To begin this part, I have chosen to use excerpts of text from initial interviews with my participants from which I have fashioned poetry. I have relied upon their words and diction whilst using repetition, off-rhyme and "connotative structures" (Richardson, cited by Ellis and Flaherty, 1992, p126 - see Chapter 1) to represent 'how they were' at the beginning of the Course. These poems are an introduction to this part and are referred to as Mystories (1).

I have also decided to use text from the students' letters, the final data collected, to complete the chapters in Part IV and bring it to an end. These appear after Chapter 10 and form Mystories (2), which demonstrate what students have made of the Course.

The title 'Mystories' appeared to be appropriate because the stories belong to the students, they reveal the students' former Selves and as such, they are no longer mysteries.

An introduction to Ben, Carol, Clare, Cathy, David, Marie, Paula and Sarah.

Mystories (1)

Ben

Past lives - the Army and Police,
A structured life of discipline and rules.
I'm married with children,
I have a bike and a car -
it depends on the weather what I use.

My mother was a nurse,
My wife was a carer,
It was expected when I was a child
that I would be a nurse or a doctor - one of the two.
So I went the opposite way, as kids normally do.

I have experience of just about everything
I want the discipline, I'll never switch off.
I have been and always will be,
Not anti-social as such, but a loner.
I prefer my own company.

Nursing is structured and ordered,
People give respect to the title.
I've got to live up to that respect.
Look at Allitt, we're all suffering because of it.
I'm taking it all on board.

The best nurses are those with experience,
The ones who have lived.
You can live and be young or you can live and be old.
Those out of school can put it on paper,
When I'm struggling with my assignments, I feel like that.

I've had my eyes opened quite a bit,
When I heard I was going to a learning disabilities placement
I was horrified.

When I heard I was going to a ward,
I was horrified.
But when I got there, everyone was so accepting,
Now I understand it.

I felt there was a lot of disorder,
Of people not knowing what they're doing.
We had information from tutors and staff
We were starting to panic and thinking "Oh Christ"
we thought we'd done it all wrong.
I feel I should call you 'ma'am'.

Carol

I applied when I was sixteen.
I went round nursing homes trying to get jobs
and I worked in a nursing home for the elderly for eighteen months.
They thought I might be too young.
Working with nurses gave me an idea
of what nurses are like to work with and what they can be like.

They were very good nurses.
I did learn a lot from them
and some of them were really good and I would like to base myself on
them.

I think you got to look out for yourself.
You just have to double check everything
and be accountable for everything you say and do; you just keep your
head down.

I felt that I was constantly watching my back.
If you tell someone you're a student nurse,
all of a sudden, "I shouldn't be smoking, or be in a pub".

I had some kind of perception of Project 2000.
I think working with old style nurses as well,
they were constantly chatting about it and I really didn't think it would
be like this.

118

So many different things.
Like psychology and sociology and I sit there and think "why?"
I've got all the books together, I just haven't opened them yet!

I think when I first started,
You just want somebody to talk to and then you start
settling down and getting to know people and you keep looking for
friends.

Everytime I thought of coming here when I was at home,
I was stood in uniform, you know, a little picture in my mind.
Why do you have to wear uniform? I think it's for identity.

This is me.
I'm not just a student nurse.
Someone said to me the other day. "all you do is hold sick bags", it
made me angry.

I've wanted to do this for years,
But you can fail me on an assignment
and that would be very difficult for me, because I'm very practical.

Clare

I went away to Africa,
(to Zimbabwe, Botswana and Namibia)
after my 'A' levels - French and Psychology.
I have an older brother, he's twenty-one.
I wanted to be in the RAF, but everyone else started applying
for university.
I hadn't really thought what I wanted to do.
My mum said "have you ever thought about nursing?"
It was scary at the interview, I knew nothing about it.
I think if I knew how hard it was going to be,
I wouldn't have done it!
I had no anxieties, because I didn't know anything.
I thought it would be rubber gloves and injections.
I pictured myself on a ward.

I feel intimidated in the large group,
I don't feel that I'm one of those people who can speak up.

(I was nineteen yesterday.)
I find it hard to see myself as a student nurse -
you don't have time to think of yourself as a nurse.
I've never worn my uniform,
I've never been on a ward.
I haven't done anything - I don't know any clinical terms.
I find the prospect of three years
quite depressing really but
because I've made this my career, I put more importance on it
I feel that I'm doing something worthwhile and serious,
like I've grown up too quick or something.
I'm glad nursing isn't what I thought it was.

Cathy

I've done lots of jobs
to fit in with family life.
I've got two children of my own and a stepson.
I didn't do 'O' levels at school, when I got married I did them.

I was a night care assistant for two years
and that helped a lot.
Talking with other nurses.
They said "I don't know why you're bothering with all that".

I was excited about it
and happy.
I read all the literature.
I expected it to be like it is, in the classroom and then on placements.

I'm thirty-two
and I've worked all the way through.
I just take things in my stride;
the more knowledge I get, the better I'll be able to do the job.

I've got a husband
and a home.
I really want to accomplish this
and really work at it; I've got my husband's support and my children's
support.

Before this
I had my own horse and did hunter trials.
But now I feel tired a lot of the time,
making sure that I make meals and things like that and making sure the
children aren't left out.

I'm easy going.
I think I'm lucky you know.
But people think it's easy for me,
so I suppose that's just the sort of person I am.

They say
"Oh you'll do it" and
"you'll be fine".
But I don't feel as confident as that.
I'm not a classic case really am I?

David

My biggest problem is money,
I have a wife, two children and one on the way.
My grandfather was looked after by Macmillan nurses,
my second child was in a special care unit.
I realised that this is what I wanted to do.

It's being able to make a difference,
I'd just been working in pubs.
I am six years out of school,
so academic essays were an anxiety.
I've been a care assistant in a nursing home.

The 'old school' nurses moaned about Project 2000,
You have to be very tactful.
I was almost thinking of not bothering,
the nurses I had seen put me off.
Like 'One flew over the cuckoo's nest'.

My life is extremely full now,
I work in a pub, I work in the nursing home.
Assignments and placements -

121

but it's great.
There's not a minute in the day that I'm not doing something.

I was expecting a lot of academic work -
I was expecting more.
I think it's a perfect balance - for me it was pitched too low.
I've got one of the biggest mouths in the group.
I was voted students' rep, so it can't be too bad.

I can't wait to get started -
it's just a stepping stone.
I want to do AIDS care, which will be big business
when I'm qualified.
I know I'm going to enjoy it.

I used to call myself a nurse when I was a care assistant.
I don't know why.
I've never been one for social standing -
I know a lot of people do it.
Status probably.

The first semester was hard,
because it was easy.
I thought, "I won't bother going in today".
and "I know how to do that".
But I found the lessons ... a great help.

Marie

I like people, I like to help people,
I think I fit in really well.
I've been told "Oh she'll make a really good nurse".
I'm a student nurse, I'm going to be a nurse.

I took the DC test and failed by two marks,
It completely put me off.
I did a Diploma in business and finance,
But I really wanted to do nursing.
Now I'm a student nurse, and I'm going to be a nurse.

I've been a nursing auxiliary,
I've worked with the elderly, children and the handicapped.
It's given me confidence to go onto the wards.
I'm a student nurse, I'm going to be a nurse.

I knew it was going to be hard,
But it feels like it's too much theory.
It's not what I expected,
But I'm much happier doing this.
I'm a student nurse and I'm going to be a nurse.

I want a job with great responsibility,
I want to go into management,
I want to be a counsellor,
I want to be a practice nurse.
I'm a student nurse, I'm going to be a nurse.

I'm very keen and confident,
In fact my confidence is blooming!
I love drama, singing and acting,
I'm not afraid to say what I want to say.
I'm a student nurse and I'm going to be a nurse.

Paula

I was living with my parents,
I have a twin sister and a brother.
She's in insurance and he's an engineer.
I went to the careers office and they told me about Project 2000,
The work sounded interesting.
(If they didn't give me the right information, I wouldn't be here.)

I had loads of worries;
Whether the others had a lot of experience,
Whether I was going to get on with everyone
(I was thinking they would be one step ahead of me.)
What if I don't like anyone?
Whether I would actually like the course,
I was hoping I would.

I expected it to be really hard work,
Like anatomy and physiology -
like my mum had said.
(When it's results time she gives me a boost.)
I don't really join in that much.
For some people it's fine, but it doesn't suit me, so.

I like the expectations put on you,
the job you do
and I like wearing uniform,
(It gives you status.)
I'm a student nurse
and I say it proud as well.

I used to be quite shy,
but learning about communication
helps you to look after yourself,
(It felt strange communicating with patients.)
You look at yourself and think,
"am I doing this and am I doing that?"

Going back home now feels really strange.
What have I actually got left there
apart from my family?
(It's made me grow up.)
I want to be a good nurse
and learn about the practical side of it, (It would make me more confident.)

Sarah (Liverpudlian accent)

I was at Manchester University doing a Business degree,
The worst thing I ever did.
No one ever mentioned nursing
Until Debbie.

(She used to come in, in her uniform and stuff,
and chatting away at night, I used to think
it wa' dead interesting.
Not like profit loss accounts and that.)

124

I thought nursing was something you were born into,
d' ya know warra mean?
I said "get lost, if someone's sick, I'm sick.
I'm not washing anyone's bum".

She said, "I think you've got the right temperament".
So I did an NVQ, went to the wards on placement,
and it wa' brilliant.
I thought, "this is whar I wanna do".

I was an auxiliary for a year.
I went from knowing nothing
to learning all the basics like pressure sores.
I was a bit frightened, but it did a hell of a lot for me.

Now, if I walk in somewhere, however bad it is,
I've got the confidence.
I remember walking down the ward in Liverpool,
this bloke had a grand mal,
I shouted dead loud across the ward.

The way I look at it,
I've been the auxiliary who the staff nurse tells
"get the bed pan",
and I've done all the basic care, like.
I wanna be able to do more.

I could use my intelligence,
do more for people.
I always said "why are you doing that" and
"what's that for"?
I used to drive them round the bend.

When I was coming down here from up North,
that was quite frightening,
even though I'm twenty-three.
Partly because I thought everyone would be younger,
D' ya know warra mean?

6 Intentionality - Comportment Toward Nursing and the Course

This chapter aims to provide an overview of the ways student participants perceived nursing and the Diploma of Higher Education in Nursing Studies course, prior to their commencement on it in 1994. I have used Heidegger's concept of 'intentionality' (p73) as a framework to illuminate the data, which is presented under sub-headings; 'Traditional images of nursing', 'Previous nursing experience', "Project 2000, what are you doing that for?", 'Academic expectations - am I up to it?' and 'I just hadn't thought - surprises at the beginning of the Course'. Material for this chapter emerged from the initial questionnaire which was distributed to the whole cohort in the first three weeks of their attendance on the Course. The questions were influenced by my historicity - during my own pre-nursing course at a further education college in 1975, it was compulsory for students to attend a chosen 'experience placement' in order to gain an insight into healthcare systems and to become familiar with hospital environments. My placement was in a physiotherapy department because the Course organisers had exhausted all their nursing placements. From their perspective I was still gaining experience in a hospital but from mine, I could not make a connection between what I perceived nursing to be and giving people electric shocks or making them ride static bicycles [I was 15 years old]. There are mixed feelings about the benefit of previous nursing experience to new recruits (see Chapter 4). I was interested to learn whether participants in my study had had any previous nursing experience, what form it had taken, and how, if at all, it had affected their transition from being members of the public to being student nurses.

Insight into the work of the nurse is of course, not the only influence upon smooth transition into the student role. Aspects of home life, peer interest in nursing and the media, all have a role to play in the way that students perceive the job of the nurse and the educational Course they undertake (Broadhead, 1983). Academic adjustment is a complex process and impacts upon all higher education students (Barker, Child, Gallois, Jones and Callan, 1991). It is a dynamic, interactive process which takes place between the person and the environment - directed towards an achievement of 'fit' which students achieve with the academic context. Understanding the ethos and expectations of higher education is an important factor which impacts upon the student's ability to 'belong'. These influences are explored in this chapter in relation to how the student participants perceived their new role occupancy. Although I have not been able to present all experiences and perceptions, my intention is to represent how different 'comportments' (Heidegger, pp161-162) provided a starting point for their journeys through the Course.

Traditional images of nursing

The Hemsley-Brown and Foskett (1999) research concerning career desirability in young people, provides alarming reading to those of us in the nursing profession who recruit nursing students based on a perceived match between personal attributes, knowledge concerning the chosen career path, expectations and the job of the nurse. They state that their sample of seventeen year olds viewed caring to be associated with self-sacrifice and the notion of being friendly, loving and dedicated were seen to be more desirable than intelligence. Nursing was perceived to offer few opportunities in terms of reaching 'the top' and had visibly low status compared with other careers they had chosen. Although nursing is thought to be highly regarded by the general public, the 'invisibility' of the knowledge and decision-making components of nursing practice contributed toward the perceived lack of status. The authors conclude that even though the education of nurses has changed significantly, the old 'apprenticeship' image of a young female nurse prevails.

Damasio (1994) believes that individuals can represent anything without externalizing it and to represent something is to form some kind of image, concrete or abstract, of that thing. If this is so, then images must be formed from memory traces of sensory experience - what I call 'experience through association'. My suggestion is that we are all able to experience what things would be like because we have images portrayed to us continuously through, for example, the media. Seeing images and having some relatedness to them through the media can result in experience through association. This could be called indirect experience, but the image is so vivid, that an individual can construe it [albeit from their own frame of reference], and thus have comportment toward any situation or phenomena. Experience through association can, I believe, be acquired through other channels. When my participants began the Course, they had perceptions of it and the accuracy of these perceptions depended a great deal upon the source of the experience through association. Sometimes they gained their perceptions from mothers who had been nurses, or from traditionally trained nurses with whom they worked in nursing homes. The senses are fed information from several differing perspectives and seeing these other aspects or dimensions of nursing and the Course, provides other 'partial perceptions' which then help the Course to manifest itself in consciousness. According to Kelly (p50) constructs may not change until an individual is exposed to a similar event or experience which forces a modification of the construct. But it appears that an individual may choose to continue to use old constructs, even if they have been exposed to more recent similar events or experiences - thus their perceptions of nursing remain tainted by traditional images. Dasein comports itself towards something possible - it anticipates a 'potentiality for Being' (Heidegger, p306) which I think, suggests that the individual is capable of adapting to unexpected situations despite using old constructs;

> Even in expecting, one leaps away from the possible and gets a foothold in the actual.
>
> (Heidegger, p306)

To 'have concern for', 'expect', 'anticipate', 'comport' and appreciate 'possibilities', in Heideggerian terms, means that we have the potential to adapt to reality and events which happen despite our sometimes distorted 'intentionality'. This immediately brings to my mind the potential for disappointment and subsequent pessimism about related events and experiences. Heidegger (p308) however, says that Dasein guards itself against 'falling back behind itself' and 'dispels danger' and also has some 'understanding of the potentiality'. The meaning I assign to this, is that in our anticipation of something, we also appreciate the negative as well as the positive possible outcomes. Although we may be disappointed that what we anticipated is not as we hoped, we are able to cope with the new situation, because of our consideration of other eventualities. We can never be absolutely certain of future experiences and therefore Dasein prepares itself for the unexpected.

When Paula started the Diploma course, she was shocked that she was not taught to take blood pressures in the classroom before going onto clinical placements. At the time of these students attending the Course, there was a strong belief that all practical skills should be learned in the clinical areas, taught and supervised by experts in clinical practice, rather than by tutors who could have been several years out of practice. Paula's expectation of being taught practical skills in the classroom is a derivative of her mother's stories, yet she claims to have read current literature regarding the Course and understands the philosophy of 'Project 2000'. She has therefore employed inferentially incompatible construction systems, and this is alluded to by Kelly (p58) in his explanation of the fragmentation corollary within his basic theory of personal constructs. Kelly asserts that even though an individual's construction system is continually in a state of flux, successive formulations may not be derivable from each other. It is possible that what Paula thinks about nursing today may not be inferred directly from what she was thinking about it yesterday. However, the old construct may be a legitimate precursor of the new construct, but Kelly argues that the relationship is a collateral, rather than a linear one. With this in mind, it is also important to understand why constructs are not derivatives of immediately antecedent ones. My interpretation is that Paula values the stories told by her mother who had undertaken some nurse training because her portrayal of nursing is from her mother's own repertoire of experiences. There is a reality about being told about experiences first hand by the experiencer. The information gleaned from leaflets and from the UKCC, although formal and perceived to be factual, does not possess the individuality and personal stamp that pervade stories of experience. These contrasting sources of personal and factual information appear to represent 'this is how it was' and 'this is how it might be'.

Marie remembered at four years old, visiting her mother working as a nurse on a ward and recalling that she felt 'at home' in the ward environment. The image of her mother in uniform was very vivid for her at the beginning of the Course, but this image faded during the first six months of the Course after which Marie said that she could not remember her mother being in uniform. She stated at this time that her mother did not have a clue about Project 2000, but that she still valued her opinion about the practical side of nursing, even though *she doesn't know anything about the theoretical side.*

Ben says very little about his mother having been a nurse which suggests that perhaps she did not have much of an influence upon his career choice. As a mature student, he may only have distant memories of his mother as a nurse. His traditional perceptions of nursing and 'nursing school' appear to be more attributed to other sources of influence, such as friends who completed the traditional nurse education programme. When he did talk to his mother about the Project 2000 course, she had retorted *it wasn't like that in my day.*

I find it interesting that students in this study chose to believe traditional nursing images over more recent ones, even when information was imparted to them through leaflets and videos for instance, which were produced by the professional body representing nursing (UKCC), reinforcing that nurses were no longer trained to be 'doers' of tasks. Perhaps there is an association with Merleau-Ponty's (1962) explanation of intentionality which portrays the concept on both a reflective and pre-reflective level of existence. He explains that reflective intentions are those of which we are explicitly aware. We are able to identify how perceptions at this level are formed; from where they originate and actually how realistic they are. Pre-reflective intentionality however, results in an individual's expression of their perceptions through action, unaware of how accurate they are. In relation to my students and their comportment toward nursing, I would suggest that their traditional images of nursing are pre-reflective intentionality, whereby their perceptions continue to be reinforced by mothers, colleagues in nursing homes and the media. After all, these images are still being supported by various people and the students had little alternative experience of any other image of nursing. Reflective intentionality however, would comprise evidence collected by the individual about the Course as it exists. This would call for some cognitive processing whereby students interpret what they have just taken in and set it against pre-existing beliefs/perceptions. If this assumption is valid, one could assume that pre-reflective intentions are more enduring and substantial than reflective intentions. Alternatively, one could consider that an individual, when confronted with the opportunity for making a choice, will tend to make that choice in favour of the alternative which seems to provide the best basis for anticipating the ensuing events. Kelly refers to this dilemma within his 'choice corollary' and states that it is the individual's choice whether they choose security or adventure (p45). In other words, we choose to believe the perception which will confirm our anticipations. The perception may be pre-reflective or reflective in terms of its intentional nature.

Those with prior nursing experience

My own experience as a nurse and a nurse tutor/senior lecturer has led me to believe that although perceptions of nursing change during the Diploma of Higher Education in Nursing Studies course, not all student nurses develop a self-concept as a nurse until the Branch Programme of the Course [or indeed, after completion of the Course in some instances]. It may be that students develop an identity within the occupational group of auxiliary nurses as a result of having had previous nursing experience and as a consequence, they develop different preconceptions and perceptions of what nursing and nursing education entails. These nursing encounters are seen as 'filters to experience' (Pilhammar-Andersson, 1993), which determine how conceptions and understandings develop in relation to nursing practice. Davis (1991) believes that previous nursing experience can hinder development of the student nurse role and that it may be necessary to break loose from existing nursing auxiliary identity before the student nurse can progress and develop a new perspective. The degree to which previous nursing experience has helped or hindered the students to perceive nursing and the Course realistically in this study, is difficult to assess. Five of the eight students had had previous experience and they had different tales to tell with regard to activities in practice and consequent perception development. Sarah had completed a National Vocational Qualification (NVQ) in healthcare and enjoyed working on the wards in a general hospital. This gave her confidence when performing *basic skills, such as bathing and lifting the patients*. She had realistic images of what nurses would be doing during her placements, but admits that she found it quite hard to detach herself from the nursing auxiliary role which she had previously occupied. The tendency to perform tasks in the auxiliary role was commonplace in students who had previous nursing experience because they felt comfortable and useful 'doing' jobs. This construct legacy may need to be refashioned so that students perform in clinical practice as student nurses and not as nursing auxiliaries. This may mean that students have to go through a period of de-skilling in order to learn the basics from a contrasting perspective. Sarah admitted that *at times I have been disorientated with my position*, implying that her nursing auxiliary role tended to be more natural for her and the security of performing tasks from an unquestioning position was easier than standing back and questioning before doing. The disorientation also stemmed from being left unsupervised by qualified staff to do basic nursing because she appeared confident and competent to do so and yet she was encouraged by tutors not to undertake activities which she had not formally been taught in college. However, auxiliary experience gave Sarah an insight into the basic needs of patients regardless of role boundaries. She demonstrated her comfort within a ward environment through her statement *I'd love a ward placement because that's where I started off and that's where I feel at home* (Sarah, one-to-one interview).

Marie had been a nursing auxiliary for nine months prior to starting the Course, in nursing homes, residential care and the private sector as well. She had also completed a pre-nursing Course ten years previously after leaving school, and believed that she had a fair insight into what nursing was about. Her expectation of the Course was that it was going to be more practical and she said that her preconceived ideas were based upon her experience of the pre-nursing course; she had been taught how to make a hospital bed and lay a tray for an enema, but confessed that the Diploma course *hasn't been anything like that*. Like Sarah, Marie believed that the experience of giving basic nursing care would give her more confidence when going onto the ward as a student nurse. During the RepGrid data collection phase, Marie realised that the pre-nursing course that she had undertaken some ten years previously had not helped her at all in perceiving accurate images of current nursing. The job had changed she said, and she had been taught things that just were not done anymore. However, her construct of nursing as a practical, task based occupation had persisted during those ten years, despite exposure to the role and nursing practice in various nursing institutions.

I recorded on my dictaphone that I thought Carol had the most accurate perception of what nursing was. I felt this way because she had commented that there was not only one personality type to suit the job of nursing, but that it took all sorts. She had worked in a nursing home for eighteen months and showed an awareness of the differences in roles and expectations of the various levels of nurse. She spoke comfortably of the realisation that she had only a limited insight into nursing, but was open to other perspectives and experiences during her placements. Despite this openness, Carol had to modify her construct of nursing during the first six months because it was based very firmly on traditional ideals and images and the Diploma course had dispelled some of those preconceptions.

David decided to work in a nursing home after he had experienced nursing as a visitor to his grandfather in hospital and his own baby in the Special Care Baby Unit of a large general hospital. He described the *psychiatric, geriatric nursing home* he worked in as not being like a hospital environment, *because it is more relaxed*. His vision of a general hospital ward environment included a busy team of nurses and frenetic pace. He did however, divorce his own perceptions from those of the general public, believing his to be more realistic. A change in his construct of nursing became apparent at the one-to-one interview when he talked of how the clients in the nursing home where he worked as a care assistant *just needed you to be there and give 24 hour nursing care.* He believed this to be in complete contrast to hospital nursing - implying that the meaning he assigned to nursing in a large institution required more acute, technical skills and knowledge. He reflected at a later date upon his feelings during a placement on a ward in a district general hospital, that he may have been advantaged over those who had not had previous experience, because he was familiar with *the seedier side - wiping bums and things like that, you know* which incidentally, also occurred in a more acute setting.

Cathy talked about her job as a night care assistant in a nursing home as *not really nursing* and yet describes getting patients out of bed in the morning and helping them with their washing and dressing. Her expectation of the job of nursing also included more *high tech* activities, such as understanding the use of equipment attached to patients. She had also had experience as a domestic in a hospital and therefore had some insight into other systems within the acute healthcare environment. Cathy thought that her role would change from being a nursing auxiliary to a student nurse and she expected giving less *hands on* care because she would be observing and everything she did would have to be overseen. In some respects, Cathy had prepared herself for the change in role by reflecting upon the core aspects of the auxiliary role in comparison to the student nurse role. This helped her to separate the perceived goals for auxiliary and student nurses. For auxiliary nurses it appears that physical care is a priority where tasks are undertaken on a day-to-day basis with routine precision. The goal for the student nurse however is to learn the role of the qualified nurse through observation, demonstration and supervision. Cathy had already identified the differences at this early stage in the Course, and yet, as will be seen in Chapter 7, she relapsed into the auxiliary role when her student 'Self' was threatened.

All of these students had had experience of giving care in nursing homes as opposed to being in the community setting or in general hospitals. It could be surmised that the experience gained pre-course by students in nursing homes is different to the environments where they perceive they will be receiving most of their nursing experience. 'Real' nursing as perceived by students, appears to take place in the more acute care settings and comprises more technical rather than the basic skills they performed as nursing auxiliaries.

Those with no prior nursing experience

Paula, Clare and Ben had not had previous nursing experience and yet it seems that their perceptions do not contrast significantly to those who had experience. Paula's mother had started her nurse training before Paula was born but had to give up because of ill health. She had looked through her mother's nursing books but stated that her mother had had little influence upon her decision to be a nurse.

Clare was unique in her anticipation of what nursing would be like. She said that she felt scared because she had no idea of what nursing was about, particularly when other students started talking about their experiences as nursing auxiliaries or care assistants. All the information she had managed to gather portrayed nursing with associated symbols of *rubber gloves and injections* and this is the clinical image of nursing that she described to me. Research conducted by Hemsley-Brown and Foskett (1999) confirms that even in the 1990s, the young people in their sample saw nursing as comprising domestic tasks and clinically related tasks such as giving an injection and passing instruments to a doctor. Despite the availability of career guidance and information from various sources including the Internet, young school leavers continue to perceive nurses as doctor's helpers where they occupy a subordinate role. Paula had also read a great deal of information about nursing and had written to the UKCC for leaflets. She had visited the careers office, but despite all this, she too had traditional images of nursing and she expected a more traditional practical course. She had expected to be disadvantaged to some extent because she did not have previous nursing experience which made her anxious about hospital ward work. Ben had no previous nursing experience as such, but had been an active member of a first aid group and in mountain rescue within the military. He described his expectations of the Course to be generally traditional, these perceptions fuelled by his mother who had been a nurse. However, he presented as a mature, keen and adaptable individual who, as a result of his varied job experiences, would respond to the challenges of nursing as a developing profession.

Students' general understanding of what nurses do appeared to derive from what they had 'seen' nurses do whilst working as auxiliaries or care assistants. This often meant that their view was task centred. Previous nursing experience confirmed this perception to some degree, because the role of the nursing auxiliary tends to be one of undertaking tasks delegated by qualified nurses and the core workforce of the majority of nursing homes is nursing auxiliaries. Despite having previous experience in a healthcare environment, an individual is as likely to misconstrue the role of the nurse as someone who has had no previous experience. This is because the physical activities of nursing are seen to be what nurses 'do', whilst problem-solving and decision-making are covert activities outside the realms of the nursing auxiliary or assistant role and are therefore not even perceived. The benefit of previous nursing experience for student nurses is the comfort and security which being able to 'do' tasks provides. In a potentially hostile, unwelcoming and unfamiliar environment, making beds, replenishing stocks and cleaning appeal because they give purpose and group membership to the new recruit.

"Project 2000, what are you doing that for?"

Sarah had a boyfriend whose sister qualified as a nurse a year before Sarah started the Course. It was she who suggested that Sarah find out about the Project 2000 course. She made enquiries, completed an NVQ in healthcare and worked on a neurology ward in a large general hospital. It appears that this individual who had completed a similar course had an influence upon Sarah's decision to start nursing;

Deb used to come in, in her uniform and stuff and chatting away at night and I used to think ... it just used to be dead interesting and we just talked for hours about it all.

(Sarah, one-to-one interview)

Conversations with someone who had completed a similar course must have provided a vivid picture of both nursing and the type of course to expect. She formed a perception based on her friend's comments about the academic side of the course;

I can remember her sitting there the night before an assignment was due in - but we could never do that at our college - and I thought that all Project 2000 courses were the same, but they're not.

(Sarah, one-to-one interview)

Sarah thought that she would be able to throw together an assignment the night before submission like Deb and pass, but she soon learned, within the first few months of the Course, that this was unacceptable and she needed to be more conscientious if she was to be successful.

Carol became very wary of qualified nurses as a result of working in the nursing home. She reported having gained insight into how nurses

135

work and emphasised how bitchy it could be. As a result of working in this tense kind of atmosphere, she observed *it's no good being a sweet loving person, but that you have to develop assertiveness and stick up for yourself* (Carol, one-to-one interview).

She refers to the qualified nurses in the nursing home as *old nurses*, meaning that they had trained in a traditional system, rather than referring to their age. Carol then, developed an impression of qualified nurses and continued throughout her first interview to emphasise the need to *watch your back, check everything you do*. She said she heard these nurses talking about Project 2000, but never became involved in the conversations herself.

The *old school* nurses described by David also *moaned* about Project 2000, but they did have an influence upon him when he first started as a care assistant. He believed that all nursing care was task orientated and that shortly before starting the Course, these 'old school' nurses nearly put him off nursing altogether. He felt that they were disrespectful to the elderly and he reported that he did not like their attitude. It appears that they only set out to satisfy the basic physical needs of their patients and this gave David a poor impression of nursing, who hoped to gain more from the Course than these nurses seemed to have acquired.

Cathy became a night care assistant, hoping that by working with qualified nurses, she would gain an accurate understanding of what Project 2000 was all about. She soon realised that they did not know much about the Course and in fact, when she showed them the Course aims and objectives, they said they did not know why she was bothering with all that. This resulted in Cathy keeping quiet about the Course, because they made her feel uncomfortable about it. The staff nurse had said to her that she thought her style of training was best and that the Project 2000 courses would not attract the right type of people who were genuinely compassionate and who could do the job of nursing. Cathy did not talk about the Course again whilst working in the nursing home because of this resistance, but inwardly felt excited and happy to be starting the Course. Both the RGNs [Registered General Nurse's] at the nursing home gave her references for the Course and she commented that *they must have said something good!*

Similar reactions to nurses being educated to diploma and degree level were captured by Hemsley-Brown and Foskett (1999), except their sample were school leavers in the employment marketplace and not traditionally trained nurses. Some young people commented that they were 'aiming higher' than nursing. One of the explanations given for this perception is that young people can see little advantage in studying nursing at university - they believe that if they are able to go to university they should try and study medicine to become a doctor which is perceived to hold a higher status. Very few occupations were seen to offer the degree of autonomy that doctors or lawyers were perceived to have which was also a factor influencing choice of career for school leavers.

Ben had a couple of friends who had been nurses trained in the traditional style. He says he expected to sit in a classroom for the first eighteen months of the Course and I would suspect that this view of Project 2000 had possibly come from them. There is the view that the balance of time is disproportionately skewed toward the academic rather than the practical aspects of nursing within the Diploma courses, a perception held by the practitioners discussed in Chapter 4.

Academic expectations - "am I up to it?"

Personal autonomy is considered to be a desirable goal in today's society (Clifford, 1999), allowing people to take some control over their lives. Boud (1991) argues that independence in learning may be the means to develop the skills required to become personally and professionally autonomous and hence self-directed or autonomous learning became one of the characteristics of the Diploma of Higher Education in Nursing Studies course. Self-directed learning is described by Hammond and Collins (1991) as a process of learners taking initiative, in collaboration with others, for increasing Self and social awareness; diagnosing their own learning needs [social and personal]; identifying resources for learning; choosing and implementing appropriate learning strategies; and reflecting upon, and evaluating, their learning. However, it is recognised that in mainstream [as opposed to nurse] education, traditional teacher-controlled curricula and didactic classes prevail and change appears to be problematic (Clifford, 1999). Some of the discussion surrounding this issue relates to the unsuitability of self-directed learning for undergraduate study, the potential of lowering academic standards and staff and student resistance.

Paula, Clare, Sarah and David studied for 'A' levels and therefore had some experience of being a student in a further/higher [mainstream] education system. However, this did not appear to prepare them for their nurse education experience. Paula did not enjoy her time at further education college and was anxious that the Project 2000 course might be tightly structured like her 'A' level course. Clare also thought that the Course would be similar to studying 'A' levels and when it was not, particularly with regard to self-directed study, she felt out on a limb;

When I was doing 'A' levels, they were small classes, rather like school in a way. It's all self-directed here, isn't it - that's quite difficult sometimes - you tend to get spoon fed at the other college and here you have to do it yourself.

(Clare, one-to-one interview)

She found it difficult to focus her studies and felt she needed more direction than the tutors were giving her. I believe that students can only have a perception of the Course or comportment in relation to it, if it has structure: structure in the way that it is organised and how content is arranged within it. Perhaps students have difficulty with self-directed learning, because they perceive it as being unstructured. This view is supported by research (Boud, 1995; Clark, 1995; McKay and Emmison, 1995) which has shown that some students resist learner-controlled learning because it demands more of their time, they doubt their ability to assess, they see grading as a staff responsibility and then feel frustrated and impotent because of the lack of structure and direction.

Within nurse education, students at undergraduate or diploma level are not yet invited to construct the content of their courses; within the institution where this study was conducted, students were only encouraged to take control of what they learned within the confines of the particular course and so it might not be considered to be thoroughly learner-controlled.

Clare also had a different attitude toward the nursing course, because she had chosen it as a career, whereas the 'A' level programme was a *means to an end*. Along with a traditional image of nurses with their rubber gloves and injections, Clare commented that she thought that doing a nursing course would be getting away from academic work and that it would be more practical. At first she was disappointed about this apparent misconception, but commented later that she was pleased that nursing was not as she had imagined.

Sarah had completed her 'A' levels and two and a half years of a business degree. She reported having a *bad experience* with higher education because she did not achieve the learning outcomes for her third year. She had found university *boring* and had obviously chosen the wrong career at that time. She talked to me at the first interview about being prepared for the academic work and that she had studied at degree level and therefore expected that the Diploma course would be plain sailing. At a later data collection phase, she admitted that there had been more work on the Degree programme, but that it had not been at such a high standard as the Diploma course. The belief that she would

138

find it easier lulled her into a false sense of security which had quite an effect upon her academic performance and confidence throughout the remainder of the Course. From a constructivist viewpoint, Sarah's anticipation of the level of academic work was inaccurate and her understanding of these levels went through a process of revision. Kelly (p51) refers to this validation and successive revision in the light of unfolding events within his 'experience corollary'. Sarah learned that her assumption about levels of academic work was inaccurate and that, despite validation and moderation processes, individual professional disciplines may have their own levels and standards. The student in this type of situation had to make efforts to realign previous experiences with the current one. By so doing, other perspectives were brought into play, such as the student's own comportment toward nursing, their own perceptions about levels, previous learning experiences, anticipated content of the educational programme and past academic performance.

> The person who stands agog at each emerging event may experience a series of interesting surprises, but if he [sic] makes no attempt to discover recurrent themes, his experience does not amount to much.
>
> (Kelly, p52)

David's anxiety about academic work stemmed from not having studied for six years. He implied in the first interview that he was ready for a demanding course in terms of the academic work. Neither Carol nor Cathy had studied at a higher level. They had both been accepted onto the Course with GCSEs (General Certificate of Secondary Education). Carol's anxieties about academic work started at an early stage when students were asked to write a diagnostic portfolio so that study skills could be assessed. She found this very unnerving because she had not given the written work much thought prior to starting the Course. This may go hand in hand with the more traditional image of nursing as a practical discipline. Cathy was not surprised at all about the amount or level of the work. She was surprised at the prescriptive nature of the assignments in terms of guidelines and topics and believed that she would be doing more project type work where she could choose what she wanted to pursue out of her own interest.

Marie had entered the Course using her B.Tec National Diploma in Business and Finance. Like Sarah she believed that if she had coped with a National Diploma, she ought to be able to cope with a nursing diploma. Marie was surprised that there was so much *in-depth sociology and psychology* and said she had not expected so much theory. Students who expect a predominantly practical course often experience

139

disillusionment at the beginning. Jowett (1995) highlights many of the reasons assigned to high attrition rates during the early Dip.H.E. nursing studies courses which include unrealistic workload and academic expectations and an imbalance between an 'impersonal' ethos of higher education and the 'approachable' college of nursing. These contrasting delivery systems were consistently described by students in Jowett's study which she states has implication for learning, levels of direction, pitching and pace of work.

Ben did not have any particular anxieties about the assignments and talked very little about the academic demands of the Course during the early data collection phases. He drew confidence from having completed an access course which prepared him to some extent for the academic demands. However, in a system which aspires to learners being in control of their learning, students have to adjust their expectation and accommodate more democratic relationships with staff and fellow students, and Ben clearly had a problem with addressing tutors on an equal basis because of his military background; *I see you as an officer and we're the non-comms. I feel I should call you ma'am.* (RepGrid).

Recent research in higher education with a sample of pharmacy students suggests that students do not enter university well equipped with the prerequisite literacy skills for successful university study (Holder, Jones, Robinson and Krass, 1999). A high proportion of students in the area where my study was conducted needed some form of intervention or remedial work as was alluded to by tutors in the focus groups in Chapter 4.

"I just hadn't thought" - surprises at the beginning of the Course

Paula was shocked when she discovered an excellent role model in practice who happened to be male. She talked to me about expecting the majority of nurses to be female and I interpreted her voice intonation and body language as implying that if there were males, surely they would not be as good at nursing as the females. What she admired about this nurse was his ability to deal with an emergency situation in a calm and organised manner.

Paula, Marie and Carol found it difficult to grasp the importance of learning about healthcare in the community at first, and believed that they were not really nursing on placements in the community setting. Again this perception originates from their image of nursing taking place in hospitals and not anywhere outside of the institutional setting.

Marie thought to herself many times during the first semester *where is all the nursing in this?* and *what's going on - what am I doing?*

I was interested in her remarks about how she could have prepared herself more for the Course if she had known more about it and then she could have *changed my views and got geared up for it.* It came as a surprise to many students that they spent much of the first couple of semesters in community placements. Carol stated that despite working in the community she could not wait to get some nursing experience. Because of her perception of nursing 'happening' in a hospital, it was unfortunate that Carol was unable to identify a good role model in her experience to date in the community. Because none of these nurses appeared to her to be doing the job of nursing as she perceived it, she was unable to transfer any of the skills the community nurses demonstrated, to the hospital setting. She therefore could not see how the community experience could be of value to her.

David discussed with me how the media portrayal of nursing gave a glamour image, especially through programmes such as 'Casualty' and 'Jimmys'. It is these 'experiences through association' that give the public their perception of nursing. Indeed, Clare said that she thought it would be like the media portrayal and that she would be in a continuously hectic environment where she would often be left alone to cope.

Sarah was surprised that there were several mature students on the Course. Before she arrived in the study area, she believed that she would be one of the oldest students at 22 years old. She was pleasantly surprised though and recognised that her perception stemmed from the image of the traditional school leaver recruit.

There is more to 'intentionality' than just having purpose

Husserl (1991) argues that the human sciences fail because they do not take into account intentionality - the way the individual mind is directed toward objects and subjects by virtue of some mental content that represents them.

> Man looks at his world through transparent patterns of templates which he creates and then attempts to fit over the realities of which the world is composed. The fit is not always good. Yet without such patterns the world appears to be such an undifferentiated homogeneity that man is unable to make any sense out of it. Even a poor fit is more helpful to him than nothing at all.
>
> (Husserl, 1991, p211)

Kelly (p7) calls these 'constructs' and believes that the patterns and templates are ways of construing the world. He believes that people strive to predict the course of events and that constructs are representations which they test against reality. Just as constructs are used to forecast events, so they must also be used to assess the accuracy of the forecast, after the events have occurred. When constructs are used to predict events or happenings, they are subject to validation and susceptible to change or revision - "we assume that all of our present interpretations of the universe are subject to revision or replacement" (Kelly, p11).

Intentionality is, for phenomenologists, an ontological concept. It is not only about perception, but includes the extraction and use of information about one's environment, which includes the senses of sight, touch, hearing, smell and taste. Perception on its own therefore is not inclusive of consciousness, knowledge and experience - intentionality is cognitively more complex than perception - it includes all these things. Perception is seen to be internalisation of the information gained by the senses, intentionality is cognitive whether we are aware of it or not (Honderich, 1995, p652).

Crotty (1996) believes that it is difficult to grasp the meanings of 'intention' and 'intentionality' because of their associations. This is because we have already had everyday meanings attributed to these words. He criticises nursing research which claims to be phenomenological in approach while bearing little resemblance to Heidegger's notion of intentionality. In the thirty pieces of nursing research which he reviewed in the early nineties, he found that only one referred to intentionality and then it was not used in its phenomenological sense. Benner and Wrubel's *Primacy of Caring* (1989) is criticised because they talk of people consciously planning to achieve certain ends and this is considered too narrow a view of intentionality. Other authors have examined intentionality in relation to communication and psychology (Manusov, Rodriguez and Scott, 1989) and the manifestation of intentionality in conscious and unconscious states (Natsoulas, 1992). May (1969) believes that intentionality is the structure which gives meaning to experience and should not be identified with intentions, but is the dimension which underlies them.

Ontologically, Heidegger (1962, p23) introduces his own term for the way human beings relate to things, verhalten, translated as "comportment". This refers to our directed activity, precisely because the term has no other overtones. He states that comportment and intentionality are not merely acts of consciousness [as with intent], but

142

of human activity in general. Intentionality is attributed not only to consciousness, but to Dasein [see Chapter 2] and comportment is not only about directing-oneself-toward, of being-directed-toward but also about perceiving and experiencing. Perceptions direct themselves toward sensations, representational images and memory residues which, in turn, give us determinations [intent] and experiences. Intentionality therefore is conscious, perceptive, affective and subjective. More recently, Anderson (1994) has presented an adaptation model of adjustment which acknowledges the interplay between emotions and cognitions, followed by actions and resulting in learning. Ultimately, Anderson proposes that an individual may understand and adjust to any situation. It occurred to me that the components of Heidegger's intentionality and Anderson's adaptation model are similar, but that Anderson's model is much less complex and can be more simply applied to everyday situations (Ramsay, Barker and Jones, 1999).

From the literature it seems that intentionality has been explored from a neurophysiological perspective, that is, how the brain processes information, and from a philosophical-psychological perspective, how the brain has semantic content, enabling it to understand. Becker (1992) describes intentionality as a natural part of human nature; "to live intentionally is to construct a meaningful life and world, both for self and others" (p25). She believes that when we intend something, we strive to make it happen. These intentions become quests for meaning in a world of objects which are solid, enduring and separate from ourselves (Ellis and Newton, 1998).

Husserl (1962) characterised intentionality as a "human meaning making activity" and thereby linked it to horizon which provides a context in which meaning is constituted.

It also appears that 'anticipation' has a role in intentionality and that the function of anticipation in an individual's directedness-toward can be detected. Interested anticipation occurs when an individual is emotionally motivated toward something and a process ensues whereby attention is directed in response to the needs of an individual. Ellis and Newton (1998) believe that there are three elements of consciousness, which include "interested anticipation", "image formation" and "activation of past afferent [incoming] data". These constitute the three temporal moments of past, present and future, so that every conscious experience seems to be stretched out over an extended interval, rather than encapsulated in an infinitesimal "present moment" (p437). In relation to 'anticipation', Kelly summarised his theory in one fundamental postulate which stated that "A person's processes are psychologically channellised by the ways in which he anticipates events" (p103). According to Kelly, when we look for something, either consciously or unconsciously, we prepare ourselves to see what it is we are looking for. We always have an anticipation, image, concept of what we are looking for or what we are about to experience or see. This appears to be a very apt premiss from which to analyse student's intentionality toward nursing and the Course, particularly as it has been suggested that students' orientations towards their learning and their conceptions, perceptions and expectations are major influences on their learning in academic environments (Akerlind and Jenkins, 1998). It was particularly rewarding to access the perceptions of my participants within three weeks of starting the Course, whilst their pre-course beliefs were still unsullied by clinical placement experience, and to talk with them after six months on the Course. This gave me an opportunity to listen to their changing constructs about nursing and the Course and these were effectively captured using a modified repertory grid technique at the six month data collection phase. I have subsequently encountered Moustakas' (1994) "summary of the challenges of intentionality", which encapsulate all my processes succinctly as follows:

- Explicating the sense in which our experiences are directed.
- Discerning the features in consciousness that are essential for the individual of objects (real or imaginary) that are before us in consciousness (noema).
- Explicating how beliefs about such objects (real or imaginary) may be acquired, how it is that we are experiencing what we are experiencing (noesis).
- Integrating the noematic and noetic correlates of intentionality into meaning and essences of experiences.

Summary

It appears that students perceived the Course in relation to what they wanted it to do for them; that is, to become a competent practical nurse. They viewed the Course therefore as an opportunity for them to refine practical skills; they viewed it as a way of learning about bodily systems as opposed to healthcare; they viewed it as a means of learning how to care for ill people and ultimately as a way of learning to work as a ward nurse. They viewed nursing through the lens of the media and they viewed it the way their parents told them it used to be. They appear to have chosen not to heed what the information leaflets say. This may be because they did not have experience, or any understanding of this 'new' way of nursing. They prefer to believe what appears familiar to them, that is the traditional portrayal of nursing and nurse education.

Using Heidegger's concept of intentionality to illuminate students' comportment toward the Course and nursing in this chapter has extended my insight into their lifeworld; I have been able to identify the influences upon them and how these shaped/structured their visions and perceptions. I have tried to convey to the reader how students had directedness-toward nursing and the Course they were undertaking and show how these manifested themselves within the students' consciousness.

Chapter 7 is concerned with the students' experiences which demonstrate their threatened Selves which can be best understood through the Heideggerian concept of thrownness.

7 Experiences of Thrownness

In Chapter 6, the student participants' comportment toward nursing and the Course were explored and it could be seen that their constructs were shaped according to perceptions and experiences which, in turn, influenced their role as student nurses at the beginning of their three year nurse education programme.

This chapter is concerned with Heidegger's (p174) concept of "thrownness" and how it has been useful in illuminating the students' experiences related to their threatened Selves. I have drawn on data from various phases to portray experiences which have had a negative influence upon students' development. I have chosen particular scenarios from the trove of student data which reveal the uniqueness of experiences, but at the same time explicate shared dimensions of thrownness. To assist my understanding of Heidegger's work in relation to thrownness, I have used the 'key to special terminology' provided by Sartre (1969, p629) in 'Being and Nothingness' to define and make usable some of Heidegger's terms and provide an approach that can illuminate the 'becoming' process. Thus my interpretation occurs not only through my own understanding, but through Sartre's interpretation of Heidegger's work. It might seem that this intricate nexus of interpretations holds the potential to provide an incomprehensible account. My counter argument would be that I have made use of Sartre's glossary when and where Heidegger's concepts fail to be useful. Therefore, what is written here remains my own interpretation.

Thrownness is a concept unique to Heidegger. It does not arise in other phenomenological approaches, yet potentially, it offers a valuable means of exploring student experience. However, as with Chapter 6, I have found that Heidegger's concepts yield greater value and hold on experience when integrated with other theoretical approaches; in this case, Sartre's work is particularly helpful.

What does it mean to be 'thrown'?

Oddly, perhaps, to understand 'thrownness' it is easier to start with the 'not thrown'. Being familiar in an environment where we are

146

comfortable amongst our own definite range of entities provides us with boundaries. It is about having power and control over the destination of 'Being' [Dasein] and confirmation that what one interprets is accurate within the given context. It is because Dasein has this certainty about some situations, that it has the potential to be thrown in others. Thrownness is one of Heidegger's "existentials" (p264) which implies that it is simply an aspect of "being-in-the-world" where we have a concept of ourselves living amongst others.

Thrownness means that being has been brought into the 'there', but not of its own accord (p329);

> Dasein gets dragged along in thrownness, that is to say, as something which has been thrown into the world, it loses itself in the world in its factical submission to that with which it is to concern itself.
>
> (Heidegger, p400)

It appears that Dasein will often be subjected to thrownness and indeed, will often be prepared for thrownness to occur, particularly in situations where Dasein has been unsettled before. Kelly (p359) explains how dimensions of a person's constructs evolve in response to "life's vicissitudes" and refers to fear, extents of anxiety, defences against anxiety and hostility as being dimensions of threat. For me, thrownness in all its dimensions involves threat to the Self, whether it be in a personal or a professional way.

Kelly believes that some people have much more difficulty than others in finding adaptive solutions to their problems in some situations but make transitions more easily in other areas. It appears that his personal construct theory acknowledges that one's core structures can be threatened by prospective change and in situations where there is abandonment of everything familiar.

As previously stated, being certain of something means that there is always the chance of that certainty being ousted; almost like experiencing a false sense of security. In thrownness, Dasein is brought face to face with unsettledness which results in the person being ill equipped to deal with a situation, usually as a consequence of not having fore-understanding or the knowledge to be able to make informed choices and thoroughly considered decisions. This in turn causes the individual to feel lost and provokes a sense of bewilderment or, at the extreme, the Self is unable to react or defend.

There were many, many examples of situations in which students felt threat to their personal and professional Selves and I had to consider carefully when I perceived the students to be really thrown, or just fazed.

I identified how being thrown was different from feeling fazed in order to detect degrees of thrownness within the students' experiences. This helped me understand the severity of the situation for the student. Being fazed means that momentarily the individual cannot make an informed decision but can go on to do so in a short space of time. Being fazed causes anxiety but not to the extent that there is psychical and physical shock. My interpretation of thrownness includes a degree of spontaneity, whereby the individual might try to rescue themself from the unfamiliar situation, or look to others to rescue them. This rescuing activity is not based upon a considered decision, rather it is a spontaneous activity to rid Dasein of immediate discomfort. Sometimes, Dasein is so lost that there is no attempt at all to rescue Self or seek the help of others, which results in the discomfort of the situation being prolonged. It is as if the Self suffers physical or psychological shock, or both. Once thrownness has been experienced in a given situation, there is the opportunity to work out possibilities, should the situation arise again. Through understanding, what was once alien, may become part of Self. The Self develops what Heidegger refers to as 'the ready-to-hand'; mental equipment which can be used.

The realisation that thrownness had more than one dimension, led to my developing a taxonomy of thrownness whereby an experience could be identified by its severity for the student, as follows, starting with the least severe;

Level 1 Unsatisfied anticipations - feeling inadequate
Level 2 Feeling fazed - bewilderment
Level 3 Considerable floundering - feelings of hostility
Level 4 Rescuing Self from thrownness
Level 5 Being rescued by others from thrownness.

I offer the following examples of students' experiences where their vulnerable Selves can be captured through an interpretation of Heidegger's thrownness.

Level 1 - Unsatisfied anticipations - feeling inadequate

Ben's Story

Dasein comports itself toward something by expecting it. To expect something is to understand it and also to await it. Through anticipation,

Dasein is always ahead of itself and this understanding projects itself upon the concerns of the individual so that things can be categorised as feasible, urgent, or indispensable in our everyday business.

Ben described how he was thrown by a change in management style within a single placement where he was allocated on two separate occasions. This change in style resulted in him being thrown, because his expectation did not match the reality. As he had had previous experience in this area, when he had been impressed with the team approach and support that he had received, the second allocation made him feel inadequate and isolated because suddenly he was in unfamiliar territory. The management style had changed, the staff were unhappy and there was little support for students. This change in the general atmosphere of the ward made staff appear uneasy and antagonistic toward each other. This resulted in Ben feeling that his anticipations were unsatisfied as he had had a very positive experience on the same ward several weeks before.

This experience demonstrates dissonance between what is anticipated and the reality which resulted in confusion, disappointment, distorted horizons and feelings of inadequacy. Being in an environment which is welcoming and supportive of students, encourages learning and develops confidence. Ben had been fortunate during his first allocation to this particular ward, at the beginning of the Branch Programme, as he had experienced an ideal learning environment. During this first allocation he was made to feel valuable to the team and described the sense of 'family' he felt whilst there. He claimed that this type of ward felt comfortable for him where, despite the democratic leadership style of the manager, no one ever abused the situation. On return to the ward, he felt that the general atmosphere had changed and that sub-groups of staff had splintered, causing tensions within the team. I have had experience of similar situations where students are used as scapegoats and messengers between one faction and another. This makes students feel uncomfortable and pressured from all quarters.

Ben noticed how client/staff relationships had become distant, with staff talking in their sub-groups, *appearing oblivious to all but the most demanding client needs.*

The descriptions by Ben, in his reflective practice portfolio, of his uncertainty demonstrate that his existing beliefs and frame of reference were not confirmed during his second allocation to this ward. Heidegger (p328) states that the "primary existential meaning of facticity lies in the character of 'having been'". Temporality quite obviously has a role to play in our expectation of what might be in the light of what has been. Temporality and thrownness are inextricably linked because -

the future, the character of having been, and the present, show the phenomenal characteristics of the 'towards oneself' and the 'back to'.

(Heidegger, p 328)

This sudden change in workplace ethos created a whirlwind of thoughts and perceptions for Ben because he had not been part of the change over time. This caused him to be paranoid, thinking that it might be all his fault that things were not the same, which in turn made him question his own competence.

Level 2 - Feeling fazed - bewilderment

Sarah's Story

One of Sarah's present tense commentaries illuminated perfectly the concept of thrownness in a situation where she was called to an emergency with the paramedics. They had been prepared to treat a patient with a diagnosis of a transient ischaemic attack [TIA]; the treatment of which Sarah was familiar. However, when they got to the patient, it transpired that he had had a mycocardial infarction and not a TIA. This came as a surprise for Sarah who had never seen the treatment or care of a person with such a condition. She demonstrated her thrownness by exclaiming *what the hell am I doing here?* Because she could not answer any of the questions fired at her by the patient's wife, her professional Self was threatened and she felt somewhat redundant. Sarah described feeling bewildered, but recognised that the situation arose through no fault of anyone in particular.

Thrownness in this instance relates to confounded anticipation and expectation and then lack of knowledge and unpreparedness. Having had experience of caring for patients with TIAs, Sarah was confident that she would be able to assist with the care of this patient. She explained that she was not worried about her role with this patient but when they arrived and the patient had obviously had a cardiac arrest, she became unnerved because she did not know how to deal with the situation. This feeling of inadequacy was further compounded by the man's wife who asked for information which Sarah could not give. She said she felt useless and unable to contribute anything to either the physical care of the patient or the psychological care of the relative. Sarah felt that there was nothing she could do to relieve the distress of the woman who continued to ask her questions and seek reassurance from her. My interpretation links Sarah's experience of her inability to cope with

150

Heidegger's concept of 'ready-to-hand'. He describes equipment that we use in our everyday existence whereby we recognise it by its function and our ability to apply it in order to utilise the function. On a cognitive level, I envisage that Sarah had the mental equipment to deal with a TIA, but not the mental equipment to deal with a cardiac arrest. The mental equipment is knowledge - and in her particular situation it was not ready-to-hand. Dreyfus and Hall (1993) claim that

> Human beings always find themselves in the midst of a world of equipmental things whose significance consists in their appropriateness (or inappropriateness) for various practical roles.
>
> (Dreyfus and Hall, 1993, p6)

If something is ready-to-hand, then it is always contextualised. That is, the user knows what the function of the equipment is and uses it in the appropriate way. In Sarah's case, she was thrown because she had knowledge [equipment] that she could use in a particular situation [TIA], but because of the change in diagnosis and subsequent care of the patient, this equipment was redundant and consequently she was fazed. What she needed was the equipment [knowledge] to be able to care for the patient with an MI and this was not ready-to-hand. Fundamentally it is about Being assigning significance to equipment that can be used in the appropriate context.

I consider Sarah's experience of thrownness to be less severe than that of Cathy [which follows] because Sarah does not talk of feeling 'paralysed' or being in a state of panic. However, for both students, the experience was relatively short in comparison to those at Level 4 or 5, in which prolonged states of discomfort and threat to the psychical, emotional and physical Selves might occur.

Level 3 - Considerable floundering - feelings of hostility

Cathy's Story

Cathy described a very common situation amongst student nurses when she arrived for her first day on a new placement. She had expectations of what she might be required to do, but the newness of the situation resulted in her being thrown in terms of the unfamiliarity of routines. She reported that she stood doing nothing and felt lost because the others went about their work apparently ignoring her; she started to panic because everyone else looked busy and this made her feel very

151

uncomfortable. She reported *I was almost paralysed; I just couldn't think of anything to do and I felt really stupid.* The lack of direction in this instance resulted in Cathy "being in the 'there' but not of its own accord" (Heidegger, p175). She added *I'm spiralling down to inadequacy.* This report of a mundane situation illuminates the emotional roller-coaster that students endure on a day-to-day basis, where thrownness is a common occurrence.

Despite the apparent simplicity of Cathy's experience, the accompanying thoughts and feelings cannot be underestimated. Because all the other nurses within this environment appeared to be going about their business, Cathy felt isolated and was tempted to revert to the nursing auxiliary role which was familiar to her. Kelly (p362) believes that when the Self is threatened, a person is likely to regress when the advantages of a new outlook are momentarily lost. By regressing into her auxiliary role, Cathy promoted feelings of security and non-threat.

Her allocated supervisor for the shift had left her alone and had seemingly disappeared. She described how the other nurses donned their aprons - a symbol that they belonged to the team, and appeared to know exactly what they were doing. She reiterated that they were all working together as a team and that it *felt like I had no place in it.* It transpired that the staff nurse had made assumptions about Cathy's abilities to *set to* and get the work done because she was a second year student. Making assumptions can result in the student being left alone without sufficient supervision, which in turn causes them to feel isolated and inadequate. Being thrown in this situation had the effect of threatening all the confidence that Cathy had built up during previous placements.

Cathy appeared not to have had the ability to transfer skills she had gained from previous placements to the ward where she felt thrown. Bobrow and Winograd (1977, p32) state that the results of human reasoning are context dependent and that the structure of memory includes not only the long term storage organisation [what do I know?], but also takes into account the current context [what is in focus at the moment?] They believe that this is an important feature of human thought, not an inconvenient limitation. Given this conjecture, I would assume that Cathy would have been able to recognise aspects of the ward work where she could have made a contribution, in the new context. But this perspective does not appear to take into account all the other subjectivites which made Cathy feel isolated and ignored.

One strong theme emerging from the data in Philpin's (1999) study of socialisation, was the nature of the socialisation process in relation to the work contexts in which nursing was experienced. Respondents often sharply contrasted accounts of experiences in 'acute' and 'chronic' areas of health work. 'Acute' nursing areas include operating theatres, intensive care units and surgical wards whereas 'chronic' areas are often represented by medical and elderly care wards. Philpin argued that nursing in an 'acute' area is medically dominated, involving highly technical interventions whereas in the 'chronic' medical wards, nursing was found to be more distanced from the medical model and patients had a more active role in their care. This being the case, it is understandable that students find difficulty in transferring skills from one practice placement to another.

Cathy made a statement about being *paralysed* in her experience of thrownness. Heidegger writes that in anxiety as in fear, Dasein is "inhibited" and "bewildered" (p395). At the limit Dasein is "paralysed" and Heidegger notes that anxiety is like darkness, since in the dark one is surrounded by "equipment" and yet is unable to use it. When an anxiety attack subsides, Dasein lets itself be absorbed back into making itself at home in the world as if the anxiety had been nothing. It appears that the 'not-at-home' is accepted as a way of Being in the event of thrownness. Cathy contemplated doing that which was familiar to her - the role of the auxiliary. Once she had tried to harness her anxiety and 'pulled herself together', she was able to rescue herself and join in with donning the apron and finding a familiar pattern of activity within the realms of an auxiliary role.

Clare's Story

Clare talked of a situation where she was in an unfamiliar ward environment when her anxiety was further intensified by a senior nurse who *had a go* at her without apparent reason. Because Clare was new to the ward, the abruptness of the encounter left her feeling shocked. This, unlike the previous three scenarios, provides a record of a student feeling thrown by a member of staff rather than a clinical situation. She reported feeling very vulnerable but unable to vent her anger at the senior nurse. Unsure of what to do after such a confrontation, she found herself floundering - level three of my taxonomy of thrownness. Clare said she felt feeble against a nurse in a powerful position and that she scurried off without retaliation. This demonstrates the student's fragility in existence - thrownness. Clare herself used the term *fragile* in describing her feelings during and after the event.

Clare chose to exit her situation immediately and turned to her supervisor who she saw as her advocate and relayed the tale to her. This episode had quite an effect upon Clare who felt angry at the time, but at a later data collection phase, said that she would not be intimidated again in such a situation. The incident was so hurtful to Clare that she was close to tears. This was her first ward placement and she had been looking forward to it. Thrownness in this context could have acted as a catalyst to decide whether she remained in nursing or not. Her description of feeling fragile captured the negativity of thrownness. I could assume that Clare took the senior nurse's comments to heart because she was already in an uncomfortable situation in the new ward environment; or that Clare felt she did not particularly belong anywhere on this first day of a new placement; or that she had no understanding of the particular dynamics within the nursing team; or that really, she did not want to be there at all, but on the previous placement where she had developed a role for herself and the people were familiar to her.

Burkitt's (1991) "structures of signification" and Heidegger's "referential whole" (p187) seem to refer to aspects of an individual's existence whereby the environment is formatted in order to make things familiar. Clare had no access to the format. This was her first ward placement and she was not aware of the cultural expectations or how the placement ethos was communicated through behaviours of others. The senior nurse's outburst may be indicative of how that collective perceived learners. For the permanent staff, all things about the practice area were familiar and they saw it for what it was and how it functioned. Heidegger speaks of; "that familiarity in accordance with which Dasein ... knows its way about ... in its public environment" (p405).

This general skill is not activated on certain occasions only; it is active all the time. In a familiar environment, we are masters of our world, constantly effortlessly ready to do what is appropriate (Dreyfus, 1991; p103). Perhaps this episode, which demonstrates thrownness, arises from the distance in horizons between these two individuals and is evidenced by Clare's unfamiliarity and the senior nurse's familiarity with the everydayness of the ward environment.

Level 4 - Rescuing Self from thrownness

Carol's Story

In her reflective practice portfolio, Carol described a situation where she was left alone to deal with relatives who had just been bereaved. The staff nurse supporting the relatives had been called away and Carol was the only nurse available to deal with the situation. This was a new experience for her and she was given the task without any warning. In her reflections, she described feeling vulnerable in a personal and professional way. Her anxieties were associated in particular with conveying to the relatives her feelings of sorrow, without compromising her professional Self. She recognised that she needed to state how she felt, but that she should also be useful to the family. Because of her discomfort in this situation, she chose to withdraw and leave the family alone. After reflecting on the event, Carol recognised that she did this because she felt so inadequate and unable to cope emotionally, rather than the reason she gave at the time, which was to give the family some privacy. She admitted in her reflections, that she was also having difficulty trying to confront her own feelings associated with mortality.

In this scenario there is evidence of thrownness being illuminated through Carol's inability to cope, the surprise of being forced into an alien situation and her fear of saying the wrong thing thereby involving her Self at varying levels. She had not met the relatives before and had little knowledge about their needs or how she should respond to them. My view is that she was jettisoned into this situation, with no time to prepare and no experience of a similar situation on which to draw. Caring for dying patients is part of the everyday practice of nurses and students are exposed to the emotional pain related to death, dying and bereavement during placements where illness prevails. There is a need for intimacy balanced by 'professionalism' and for advanced communication skills. Dealing with the emotions of relatives is often the most challenging aspect of caring for terminally ill people. However, students are often deprived of the experience of observing expert counsellors in action because of the very private and delicate nature of the situation. This results in students being unprepared when the opportunity arises to offer support to relatives in the event of a person's death. Carol's experience of being expected to cope, in the absence of the staff nurse, exposes an expectation that students will know how to respond, even if they have received little or no instruction. Carol commented that she felt vulnerable in a personal and professional way and it is my interpretation that she merged these two aspects of Self, because she was unable to distinguish between the two, due to her lack of knowledge. In this instance, her professional Self had no advantage over her personal Self. Her personal Self had as much idea about managing the situation as her professional Self. This merger of Selves has no conflict, rather they blur so that the individual draws upon any available resource. If there is no experience base upon which to draw, it appears that the only option is to withdraw from the situation which is causing discomfort. Carol's personal Self is represented by her need to convey sorrow to the relatives. Her lack of knowledge exposed the inadequacy of her professional Self because she did not know when

155

this might be appropriate or how her sympathies should be conveyed. She did demonstrate an awareness of the role of the professional Self though, by recognising that she should be offering support to the family and satisfying their needs. Remaining unobtrusive, whilst giving the appropriate information, is a skill which is learned through repeated observation. Carol acknowledged that she could have *let the family down* at a most tragic time and this further compounded her feeling of inadequacy. She admitted to having difficulty coming to terms with mortality and realised that there was potential for her to become emotionally fuelled by the situation. She began to think of how she would have felt in a similar situation; if it were her father who had died and how she would be feeling. These emotions created conflict between her personal and professional Selves, where both were in need of recognition. Within this one scenario, there is evidence to suggest that personal and professional Selves may merge or conflict, but in response to different demands or stimuli.

The student experience of dealing with death and dying was not addressed in the research funded by the ENB which aimed to identify perceptions of the philosophy and practice of nursing (Macleod Clark, Maben and Jones, 1996). However, there is ample evidence within their work to suggest that students are still expected to 'learn through doing' and that they do not always have the opportunity to observe the skills which they need to acquire. Indeed, their research identified that students were gradually socialised into the professional role of the nurse by perceiving and assessing them more as a worker than a learner as the Course progressed (p108).

From a social constructionist position, it could be argued that feelings and indeed, all emotions, are structured by the way we understand things. Carol exited a situation where she felt strong emotional feelings, but was unable to channel these in the appropriate manner dictated by or expected by her nurse colleagues or the culture in which she was working.

> Feelings are thus bound up with stories, myths and conventions of culture which guide people on how to react in different circumstances.
>
> (Stevens, 1996, p236)

Rosaldo (1984) suggests that certain kinds of emotional expression and ways of understanding emotions become habitual and characteristic in a cultural group. My own experiences in nursing practice regarding death and dying, include expectations by junior and senior nurses that one's own personal emotional state should not, on the whole, be evident in nursing practice. It may be interpreted as a loss of self-control and an inhibitor to professional practice. It is debatable whether Carol responded to her situation where she was faced with grieving relatives in a personal or professional domain. She may have felt that it would be culturally unacceptable for her to become emotionally involved with relatives, or that on a more personal level, she was unprepared to face the consequences of being left alone with them. Conflict or fragmentation of Self can occur as a result of confrontation or, in my descriptions of the students' stories, as thrownness where they are confronted by simple or complex situations which cause the personal and professional Self to be fragmented. Carol's response to her particular experience could be regarded as an attempt to rescue herself from thrownness - the fourth level in my taxonomy referred to at the beginning of this chapter.

Death of course, is the inescapable fate of all human beings and also features as one of Heidegger's 'existentials'. It appears from his text (pp285-311) that he is obsessed with "the end of Dasein", "the ontological analysis of death", "the structure of death" and "being-towards-the-end". The student participants in my study conveyed many experiences related to death or the dying days and hours of their patients/clients. It appears from their stories that the agents of control in clinical nursing practice provide difficult experiences and trials which they, as novices, have to undergo in order to emerge as 'expert'. Holloway and Penson (1987) believe that these experiences are part of the socialisation procedure for new members of the profession and can be paralleled with 'culture shock', whereby novices are exposed to the rituals and traditions of nursing practice. Although many occupations use the strategy of culture shock, in nursing it does not come after a lengthy process of induction to principles, theories and practice, but may happen in the very early stages of the Course. It may mean that the agents of control can change and disrupt practices fostered by those in education. Students may be confronted by the death of a patient/client on their first day in nursing practice.

Marie's Story

Marie referred to the first entry in her reflective practice portfolio where she described being *thrown in at the deep end*. Taken in its most primordial sense, thrownness in this instance refers to the student's feeling of being out of her depth and unable to cope. Similarly to Carol, on her first day of rostered service in the second year of the Course, Marie was asked if she wanted an opportunity to gain experience in counselling. As she was eager to make a good first impression, she agreed and was directed behind curtains where three relatives of a recently deceased patient sat sobbing. The relatives were distraught at their recent news and Marie talked of the discomfort of being thrust into the situation without any prior warning. She had no information about the patient, the relatives or any of the circumstances which confronted her. She had never been on the ward before and did not know her supervisor. Marie reported that as a result of her being pushed into this situation, her self confidence *took a dive* and she felt ill prepared to deal with the situation. There was no one around to offer her any support. It is apparent within her story, that the relatives felt her growing tension and began to ask her questions about her training in order to make her feel at ease. This in turn, made Marie feel emotional because they were showing care and compassion for her even in the depth of their own grief.

Thrownness in this instance related to unpreparedness, inadequacy, lack of choice and guilt. This is a similar story to Carol's where, despite the good intentions of the staff nurse believing that it would be a good opportunity for the student, the effect of finding themselves in such an emotionally loaded situation could have resulted in disaster, for both students and relatives. Dealing with bereaved relatives, without support, is not a suitable opportunity to gain counselling experience. Part of Marie's embarrassment came from having no information about the patient, which she had to admit to the relatives. From her own analysis of the situation it is apparent that she felt unable to accommodate the needs of the relatives by simply listening; although listening enabled her to gather her thoughts and then make a swift exit to make the relatives a cup of tea. In effect, she rescued herself from this potentially damaging situation, although the relatives had also rescued her primarily by initiating conversation and relieving the tension.

This whole scenario evolved out of a desire to be seen as worthwhile and to be accepted into the ward team. I have been made aware through all my participants' data that they have a yearning to belong and would, therefore, do anything to 'please' their qualified colleagues. Fear of non-acceptance and isolation of students from their qualified colleagues served as a prompt to take risks with patients and relatives. Marie, on reflection, recognises that a more suitable line of action would have been to refuse to take responsibility in such a situation and request to observe the staff nurse in the counselling role. This would have enabled her to work through some of the outstanding issues which she felt ill-prepared to tackle.

Paula demonstrated thrownness during an intimate caring relationship with a patient whose diagnosis had not been confirmed. Prior to her days off, she had developed a rapport with a man who reciprocated her friendly, caring and humorous gestures toward him. There are inevitably patients whom we all remember as being special and this was one for whom Paula felt an affinity. She reported that communication felt comfortable and free with this man and that she had grown to like him as he valued her presence. Returning from her days off, Paula learned that her patient friend had been diagnosed as terminally ill with little time to live. This came as a shock to her, but she plucked up the courage to talk to him, which she thought he would respond to positively. Her assumptions were wrong and he became hostile and threatening toward her. This resulted in Paula feeling devastated that she had lost John's trust, inadequate, uncomfortable and unsure of how to respond. Subsequently their interactions spanned less and less time as her current and following shifts progressed.

As with several of the other students' reflective scenarios, Paula chose to reflect upon a situation involving the grief which accompanies a patient dying. I believe that patients often see students as transient, more like themselves, than as one of the permanent workforce. Because of this they feel able to relate to them more as an advocate. After the news of his impending death, John became hostile toward Paula who was surprised and hurt by his unexpected behaviour. She reported a difference in his body language in that he appeared withdrawn and solemn. He was reluctant to communicate with her, feeling perhaps that he had lost his control over the situation, but that she had maintained hers. He exclaimed that she knew nothing about his illness because she was only a student. This made her feel even more inadequate. By saying that she was only a student, he had belittled the very characteristic which appealed to him in the first instance - her naivety. Paula believed that because they had developed a rapport she could offer him support as a nurse and a friend. Her self-rescue strategy was just to walk away. She felt too hurt and disregarded to stay and communicate further. The behaviour of the patient made her back pedal and she lost confidence in facing him. She admits to losing her composure and this threatened her ability to cope.

Heidegger describes the animosity of "being" in the light of "idle" talk. My interpretation of 'idle' in his text is simple conversation with others. It does not have to have a negative connotation. He says that idle talk dominates the being-with-one-another.

> The other is proximally 'there' in terms of what 'they' know about him, what 'they' say in their talk about him, and what 'they' don't know about him. In primordial 'being-with-one-another', idle talk first slips itself in between.
>
> (Heidegger, p211)

This sentence simply describes how individuals assign meaning and inference to the talk of others. John was keeping an eye on Paula to see how she would comport herself following his bad news. He may have felt disadvantaged in that she was an accessory to the 'idle talk' and responded as 'they' - trying to help, placate and reduce his anxiety.

> Being-with-one-another in the 'they' is by no means an indifferent side-by-sideness in which everything has been settled, but rather an intent, ambiguous watching of the one another, a secret reciprocal listening in.
>
> (Heidegger, p219)

Heidegger makes a distinction between "for one another" and "against one another" (p253). My understanding of this statement, is that whilst people show an allegiance to one another, there are always other dynamics operating and each individual has their own agenda. It could be construed as a self-protection strategy whereby, in the face of any disturbance, one can defend their position against the 'other'.

Level 5 - Being rescued by others from thrownness

David's Story

David described a situation where he was asked to take a client in a mental health setting, for electro-convulsive therapy [ECT]. There were several aspects of the routine care that he did not understand and there were no explanations forthcoming from the qualified staff. He had been allocated this responsibility and was left alone to escort the client. An example of his not understanding the routine care for such a procedure is his statement *she is taken out of her own bed early in the morning, just to be put into another one*. Both he and the client were left, without explanation, in a small waiting area which he described as *claustrophobic*. He was ushered into the suite by a *scary-looking* nurse who he claims also has the reputation of being scary. This further heightened his anxiety in a situation where he felt out of his depth and unprepared for what would happen. It was unchartered territory for both of them. He was then told to stand at the end of the room, which further isolated him from the only familiar thing to him - the client. In the present tense commentary in which this episode was disclosed, David used short sentences to give poignancy to the event. He said he felt useless, described his inadequacy and how he felt anxious about the situation into which he had been thrown. This was an unusual position for David, who normally oozed self-confidence. He talked about the doctor and the nurse being powerful, because they knew what to expect, and he did not. There is evidence of intimidation of both client and student, and David recognised that lack of knowledge led to his frustration - *she is very confused and so am I*. This type of oppression of the most vulnerable has been identified in the work of White (1996), who found that participants in his research were pressurised as a result of socialisation into a system whereby demands are made upon individuals which are accepted as part of the norm. He links this to the work of Habermas (1987) and talks about critical social theory and how institutions oppress the workers. He argues that the system is "self supporting" and able to generate compliance to its structures through the use of powerful socialisation processes that punish the unsure, "the poor actor in the game". The punishment is indirect in that the actors punish themselves for not measuring up to expectations. White developed a theoretical framework from a repertory grid analysis of six newly qualified nurses to identify the feelings they experience in clinical practice. Amongst the themes that emerged from his data were "feelings related to the threatened self". He implies that although anxiety is normal when working with people, there is also anxiety which arises out of a feeling of "not being quite sure of what might happen". White believes that this is healthy and worthwhile. However, he identifies the other extreme where the nurse has been thrust into an impossible situation and is expected to cope. His analysis of the grids suggests that there were situations, in which his subjects found themselves, which resulted in them feeling very stressed. White concludes that such extremes demonstrate the potential danger to the neophyte nurse. His participants appeared at times to experience situations that were beyond their capabilities; they also suggested that this type of situation is not unusual.

In David's experience, thrownness was due to unfamiliarity, preconceptions about ECT, expectation and lack of knowledge. David's scenario is laden with expectation and lack of fore-understanding. Prior to the event, he had been subjected to gossip about how *scary* the ECT suite nurse was and this description provided a menacing image to an already potentially gruesome procedure. The media have portrayed ECT in films and documentaries, where electric shocks are administered as punishment, so that it has a reputation for being sinister. David's anxiety was further heightened by his lack of understanding of the procedure and his role within it. No one had taken the time to offer an explanation about what he should expect, resulting in him being unable to give any information to the client who would have expected this of him. He perceived his role to be client comforter, a familiar role for a student, but this was taken away by the nurse who ordered him to stand at the back of the room. The student and patient were distanced and the discomfort and isolation are further compounded by David being instructed to move because he was standing in front of the clock. He demonstrated an awareness of the vulnerability of his client, stating that he was the only person available to comfort her. David remarked that no communication was forthcoming from the nurse or the anaesthetist and he was therefore unable to be an advocate for his client. This scenario illuminates an instance where a student felt unable to rescue himself or his client leading to prolonged discomfort, which could not be relieved until he returned to the ward where he could seek support. My interpretation of David's experience is that he was unable to deploy a rescue strategy in his predicament because he was rendered powerless and lacked the knowledge to be able to act. This might therefore be considered to be the most extreme and severe degree of thrownness, where he had to wait for explanations, support and rescue from others when he returned to the ward. However, the whole scenario felt like a conspiracy to him, where even the ward nurses 'sent' him into this impossible situation.

It appears that we are always being thrown into a kind of being that we already understand to some degree, like a fish in water (Nelms, 1996, p372). And yet we also live a kind of being which we can only more fully come to understand, though never completely, through our living it. Our struggle is to try, in some way, to make the world our 'home' and to try and feel comfortable with our being-in-the-world.

It could be said that each of my participants, in telling their stories where they had felt thrown, were 'homeless'. David was certainly not at-home in the ECT suite; Marie, Carol and Paula talked of their feelings of inadequacy and apparent lostness in their attempts at caring in situations related to death and dying. Ben thought he would be 'at-home' in the ward where he had had a previous placement, but found that this was not the home he had prepared himself for and Sarah thought she would be at-home with the experience when she was out with the paramedics. Clare and Cathy tell of their not-at-home experiences on new wards.

Summary

In this chapter, I have tried to elicit the uniqueness of the students' experiences which relate, within my interpretive mode, to the common theme of thrownness using a taxonomy which I developed during analysis of the data. It appears that thrownness relates to those experiences where students have been suddenly exposed to situations which unnerve them which, even at the least severe level, makes them feel inadequate and unprepared. This results in feelings of exposure. That is, their emotional, physical and intellectual Selves become vulnerable at a time when they are least expecting it.

Thrownness appears to complement the understanding of people as 'active subjects'. As people mature [personally or professionally], they become active members in a life formed by factors outside their control. The incidence of being thrown then, is more likely to occur in later adult life, because one already has a frame of reference from life experience. It is only when one has a frame of reference, or expectation, that one has the potential to be thrown from it.

I should also acknowledge the possibility of there being other levels of thrownness, for instance Level 6 could be a threshold where a student is so 'thrown' that the threatening experience is a catalyst to leaving the Course. I might also assume that, as all students experienced a degree of thrownness, it is not a concept related to a particular gender or age group.

Whilst we encourage encounter of unfamiliar situations and interaction in difficult circumstances in nursing, as educationalists, practitioners and researchers we ought to recognise that thrownness is a real issue to neophyte nurses. We should also recognise when an individual requires support and the level at which it is needed. Perhaps individuals would benefit from exploring rescue strategies which could be employed in potentially difficult situations.

Having explored students' experiences through the concept of thrownness, Chapter 8 reveals the contexts in which students find themselves 'Being-in-the-world-with-others' and how these experiences assist or retard their progression toward the desired professional Self.

8 Being-in-the-World-with-Others

The focus of Chapter 7 was the nature of students' experiences discussed in terms of the Heideggerian concept of 'thrownness'. Individuals testified to having been exposed to situations in clinical nursing practice which made them feel inadequate, fazed, bewildered and thrown. Particular experiences were selected from the data to demonstrate the taxonomy of thrownness I developed during the original, tentative analysis of the scenarios which helped me understand the meaning and severity of the experience for each student. As being thrown almost always occurred as a result of interacting with others, it may seem illogical to present a chapter about thrownness prior to a chapter about being-in-the-world-with-others. I have chosen to do so because thrownness occurred, in the main, in the early semesters of the Course, whereas being-in-the-world-with-others, is a theme which can be identified in students' stories throughout the Course.

This chapter is concerned with experiences of my student participants as they encountered others in their lifeworlds and the contexts in which they found themselves being-in-the-world-with-others.

What is 'being-with'?

To remind the reader, Heidegger assigned the word 'Dasein' to describe the nature of human existence - it implies that the world and the individual cannot be separated and indeed, translated Dasein means 'Being there' [Dasein has been described in more detail in Chapter 2]. To try to understand people from this perspective means that they must always be situated within their environment and the context in which events that affect them occur. Within environments and events the individual is always part of a network of relationships and therefore they cannot be divorced from the influence that these have upon them. Being-in-the-world-with-others forms an integral part of all the experiences conveyed to me by students in this study. Whether the 'others' were clients or patients, peers, clinical colleagues or teachers, friends and family; significant others have had a role in the 'becoming'

164

process from student to qualified nurse. Becker (1992) believes that even when alone or in isolation, an individual can still be viewed in relation to others; as a daughter or son, a victim or persecutor for instance.

Heidegger (p58), writes about different types of 'being-with'. As individuals, we can be 'for or against' another, 'with or without' another, 'passing one another', 'matter' to one another. We can show interest in one another, consideration for one another, we can empathise with one another and relate to one another. All these types of being-with involve some kind of concern for one another. Even if we do not relate, empathise or show interest in one another, we are still, by negation, not showing concern for, or they are not mattering to us. However, just because we are there, does not mean that we are 'with' others. This implies that physical presence alone is not a sufficient condition for being-with.

I have been able to identify four distinct areas where 'being-in-the-world-with-others' is exemplified; namely in students' talk about accommodation; about cliques within the main student group; in their writing about supervisors and supervision and also in episodes where they had significant interactions with patients/clients [as in Chapter 7]. As 'being-with' is a fundamental aspect of nursing, I have chosen examples to illuminate their common experiences, despite the uniqueness of each experience. This chapter is arranged in four sub-sections; 'In the Midst of Nursingness - Living-in, Moving-out', is concerned with students' stories about living in nurses accommodation; 'The Student Cohort - Them and Us' describes mature and young students' perceptions of each other; 'Being-with Patients/Clients/Relatives - Personal Investment of Self' examines how students invest their energies in caring and – 'Experiences of Learning in Clinical Practice: Being-with Supervisors' shows how students relate to their supervisors and how they identify positive and negative experiences of supervision.

In the midst of nursingness - living-in, moving-out

From my own horizon, living in hospital accommodation as a student nurse gave me a sense of belonging to an institution and living the student nurse role. My entire social and working lives were intertwined and revolved around this role. My first night in student nurse accommodation was a lonely one and I can remember 'phoning my father to come and fetch me. We were not allowed any visitors and there were bars at the windows. At that time, this commitment of

165

predominently young female school leavers meant that the outside world could not easily permeate the hospital world.

Goffman's (1968) theorizing about institutional life suggests that hospitals are powerful institutions where staff are subjected to various formal and informal rules and regulations which shape their behaviour. Neophytes to nursing are likely to experience different power relations in the hospital, education establishment and nurses home, each with their distinct cultures and practices. Once the initial feelings of home-sickness and isolation began to fade, a sense of belonging, family, trust, initiation and purpose emerged for me. If I wanted to be alone, I shut my door. If I wanted company, I opened it. I was sixteen.

Because of my generally positive experiences of living-in, I had a tendency to believe that those who did not missed the support resulting from friendships fostered in the nurses home. However, I now recognise that living-in may not be an option, or indeed a desire, of many mature students who undertake current nursing courses because they already have established homes and families. Those without homes in the College vicinity had the option of living-in and tended to accept the offer of accommodation during the first few months of the Course until they became settled in the town and found private accommodation for themselves. During the fieldwork for this study, student accommodation was provided by the NHS Trusts but was the same as in my day; sparse, stark and unwelcoming. Living in close proximity with others meant that individuals had to learn to be tolerant of each other and when this did not happen, havens were sought elsewhere. Eating, drinking, sleeping, working and socialising focused around the one thing that all inmates had in common; nursing.

Sarah moved to the area from 'up north' where she had lived with other friends and had also spent some time at boarding school. Despite her parents living fairly close to the College, Sarah preferred to live-in because she wanted to get to know people and make friends. She described the support systems available in the nurses home and how three of them were always there for each other in times of crisis - crises were usually related to the academic demands of the Course. Living at close quarters with other students also raised individual awareness about future stages of studenthood; what to expect and how difficult assignments were perceived to be. Sarah believed that this could *put the frighteners on you* and that sometimes, returning to peers in her own cohort provided the sense of levelling required to sustain the immediate semester requirements. Laing (1993) believes that 'gossip' is a group-binding, boundary-maintaining mechanism which affirms alliance and helps to establish roots. This, in turn, could help preserve the social

166

status of members in the nurses home with a view to reinforcing unity. However, Sarah moved out after about a year-and-a-half because she *just couldn't handle it.* She reported during the RepGrid encounter, that she was much happier since she had moved out to live with other members of the cohort. There had been problems with the accommodation and several students had gone to the College for support from tutors, but had been disappointed with their attitude because they did not, or would not, get involved in students' domestic circumstances. These students appeared to expect support from the tutorial staff which may stem from the belief that living-in meant that the college had some responsibility for them.

For Paula, living-in was the focus of her anxieties during the early months on the Course. She felt that it would be good to live in the *halls* because everything could centre around nursing. I was intrigued by her term 'halls' because it is not a word used in nursing to describe the nurses home. I suspected that it was a term she picked up from her brother or friends at university. The term is synonymous with academic institutions and I had visions of high ceilings, large windows and the Dickensian spirit of the 'boys as boarders'. Paula opted to live-in so that she could get to know everybody, but after 6 months realised that *all the time everything you hear is about nursing - you can't get away from it.* It appeared that living-in was a constant reminder of the job and that it became a way of life which in Paula's case was *sickening*, and she too decided to move out after a year-and-a-half. Having discussed accommodation with a couple of participants in the study, I began to wonder whether a year-and-a-half was a significant time period after which students felt they needed to move out. The specialist branches start after eighteen months of the Course and this may have been an opportune moment to change their personal and social life so that they became more autonomous and free of one of the 'ownership' dimensions of the College. Paula commented that since moving out, she was able to maintain life outside nursing and she had developed new friendships with people who were not nurses.

Living-in however, appeared to give students relatedness. Heidegger refers to "being alongside" (p80) which in this instance implies that an understanding, an empathy, a linking between individuals resulted from residing together. Students seemed to need this relationship with their counterparts at an early stage in the Course and they talked about the support systems associated with living-in and the accompanying annoyances; indeed Lum (1988) claims that informal interactions with fellow students is a powerful mechanism in promoting a sense of belonging.

Moving away from home was also Clare's main concern about the Course. As one of the youngest participants in the study, she was anxious about meeting new people and not knowing anyone. At the one-to-one interview after six months, she conveyed to me how advantageous living-in had been; it had given her a head start because she got to know people in the group and also had the opportunity to discuss work and gain support. She felt that they were *all in the same boat* and were mainly similar in age, all experiencing life away from home for the first time. The nurses home provided a secure place where support and reassurance could be obtained, but where little else apart from nursing was discussed. However, Clare said at the time, that she was enjoying her independence from family. Six months later at the RepGrid encounter Clare worked her way through the grid and started reflecting upon moving away from home. She became agitated but quiet and her body language suggested that all was not well with her accommodation. She confided that although she felt settled in the area, she missed home more than ever and this had become an issue for her. She paused to consider the consequences of telling me her plight. I asked if she was unhappy. With this prompt, Clare burst into tears and I offered to turn off the taperecorder and resume the conversation later. The tape was paused for half-an-hour during which time we had coffee and talked about possible action she could take to alleviate her apparent unhappiness in the nurses home. It transpired that living-in had become very uncomfortable for her and, though she was miserable, she could not afford to move out. The situation was taking its toll on her concentration and she was afraid that her coursework might be affected. She said that the most distressing aspect of living-in was the total lack of privacy. Heidegger (p162) recognises that in living everyday with others, individuals must constantly be concerned with how others are in relation to them, and conscious of the way that they react to, or involve themselves with others even if they do not seriously "count on" them. We are environmentally concerned because they are there and "Dasein is absorbed in the world of its concern" (p162). He believes that such being-with-one-another has the character of 'distantiality', which suggests that although students live closely together within the confines of a building, they should be able to stand in 'subjection' having the option to share being-with or being-without, although Heidegger states that "everyone is the other, and no-one is himself" (p165), implying that distantiality operates on a superficial plane. He does however, discuss elements of 'publicness' which involve an acceptable level of sharing between people, communicated within relationships and the reality of any situation.

168

I interpret distantiality occurring as a result of an individual's primary socialisation in relation to common courtesies and ability to negotiate. I think being-with is achieved through refined skills of interaction and awareness of Self, power dynamics and boundaries. It appeared that Clare was unable to deal with relationships in the nurses home because of her apparent lack of assertion and timidity in situations where other, more dominant, individuals carried her along with the tide of their decision making. This made her feel coerced and unrepresented and, to some degree, bullied. She had decided to change the situation and had, at the RepGrid stage, already made plans to move out. Her distress though, whilst telling me about the misery of living-in left an impression on me. I felt close to Clare whilst she told me about the problems she was experiencing in the nurses home. I later recorded on my dictaphone-

Clare is devastated about the situation in the nurses home. She appears really vulnerable at the moment - how much can I help her? Is it my role to help? In effect, what can I do anyway? It's all part of growing up and she needs to assert herself.

(Dictaphone, March 1995)

I was beginning to develop a protective role toward Clare and recognised that this would not be beneficial to either of us. After this RepGrid encounter, I decided that I would ask how things were if I bumped into her in College, but would not go out of my way to become involved in the intricacies of her living-in, moving-out. Feuds in the nurses home arose from an incompatible basis of expectation - lack of privacy, overstaying one's welcome, insufficient space and invasion of privacy through noise, are problems which I have been alerted to, not only by the students in this study, but by others throughout my time as a tutor.

Carol also had anxieties about leaving home and moving into the nurses accommodation. She appreciated that everyone in the nurses home would be similarly affected, a perception found by Bradby (1990) in his study of traditional students who reported sharing the good and bad times in order to gain support. Carol also found that students in more advanced semesters helped her out with books and made her feel at ease. She said that there were always people around;

I suppose there are disadvantages - You've got one room and a lot of people together so you get on each other's nerves and it's like sometimes you just want to shut the door and say I just don't want to speak to anyone. I just want to be left alone. You go to the shower and

169

*you haven't got a front room to walk into and it's just the little things -
the fridge always smells and it really does get you down after a while.*
                                        (Carol, one-to-one interview)

Obviously Carol was missing the comforts of home and feeling
frustration at the proximity of other students when trying to attend to
personal needs.

Although authors recognise the need for nurses homes to be a safe
haven for students, they appear to assume low priority with NHS
management (Plant, 1993) and continue to be a low resource concern
(Keighley, 1990), attracting problems such as theft, attacks on residents
and poor communal facilities for laundering and socialising (Tattam,
1990).

Carol also made clear how other students were not always
considerate;

*... trying to study and there's stomping up and down the corridor and
you want an early night and nothing settles down until midnight and
you just doze ...*
                                        (Carol, one-to-one interview)

Living-in for Carol reinforced her purpose for being-there;

*there are more disadvantages than advantages of living-in, but I really
do feel that I've got my identity ... you are a student nurse.*
                                        (Carol, one-to-one interview)

She also conveyed the difficulty of mixing with students who were
not living-in and this made it difficult to make friends 'outside'. Getting
out and going for a drink with friends outside the nurses home made a
change from being-with the same people. She reported;

*I eat, sleep and breathe nursing at the moment..living in the hospital,
living in the students' accommodation ... and it's always the same. You
really need to get out.*
                                        (Carol, one-to-one interview)

At the RepGrid encounter Carol reported that she too had moved out
of the nurses home into private accommodation with some other
student nurses. This was seen to be more conducive to leading a normal
life in that there was support there if she needed it from her peers, but
she could lead a life of her own away from nursing.

In her summary letter at the end of the Course, Carol wrote;

Honestly, there were times on the Course where my life felt like it revolved around hospital wards, the library at college and being locked away in the bedroom studying furiously, while secretly longing to watch Eastenders.

(Carol, summary letter)

Marie believed that living-in the nurses home was very good because it enabled students to get together and share ideas. It also gave them an opportunity to *stress out* together and compare notes with other students in various semesters. She too found that the lack of privacy was a problem and that her room was always scattered with books and a tendency to *work, work, work.*

The knock-on effect of an individual student's hysteria was evident in a description in which Marie portrayed the anguish of a student who had failed an assignment. She said that she could hear the cries and screams of this girl and she really did not need to hear it.

You get different stories from students and you think "Oh God, I wish I was in another house." You know, there are fifty students living-in a house and it's all nursey, nursey, nursey and you just can't get away from it sometimes. You just want to mix with other people from different jobs and that's the only thing.

(Carol, one-to-one interview)

The intensity of emotions and frustrations within the nurses home was illuminated by the students' stories about anxieties related to academic work and these were fuelled by students in other groups. Idle talk and gossip appeared to have been driven by students' curiosity about assignments and what to expect as the Course progressed. The need to know what comes next surpassed their need to self-preserve through ignorance. Students were often caught in the 'hype' of the gossip wave in the nurses home and this led to intense anxiety, frustration and confidence troughs. Six months after starting the Course, Marie also reported missing home, but at the RepGrid encounter this no longer applied because she had moved out of the nurses home. She was enjoying her own space and some peace even though, she said, the move had created more problems with other members of her cohort.

I began to fit some of the pieces together - snippets of stories relating to unhappiness in the nurses home and various other stories about accommodation and realised that some were linked. It is not necessary to make those links explicit here, especially as they involve several participants in this study. Suffice to say, I was intrigued by the fact that students were talking about other students and they all had a direct association with this study.

The three students who lived out were married with families of their own. On commencement of the Course, David had two children and the third was imminent. He perceived that students living-in would view him as being more responsible. However, he appeared disappointed that there were few opportunities for the group to mix and go out together and told me about an occasion organised for the group when only ten people turned up. He said that the group was a bit boring, that he had no problems with living-out and took segregation from the group in his stride.

Cathy believed that the greatest advantage of living-out was financial, claiming that she would never be on the breadline because her husband earned a good wage. She gained reassurance from her husband and children early in the Course that her goals could be achieved. Her children continued throughout to give her positive feedback, although her marriage dissolved during the latter stages of the Course. At first, I thought that she would not experience the same motivation and stimulus at her home in contrast to the nurses home. This of course, was a ridiculous assumption, given that she was, at the outset, amongst people who really wanted her to succeed despite them not really understanding the intricacies of the Course, as say, her peers would. Cathy believed that the benefit of living-in nurses accommodation included the opportunity to talk with others who had been through previous semesters and gaining advice. Senior students were perceived to be a useful resource in the nurses home who could *explain things which some junior students may be finding difficult*. She balanced this with the disadvantage of noise levels in the nurses home and the frustration of trying to study when something is *constantly going on*.

In contrast to all the other participants in this study, Ben moved-in having originally lived-out. During an early data collection phase, he believed that living-in meant that interaction with others in a similar position could be maintained and information was passed on readily. He also recognised that this was not always good for him personally and confessed that he needed to be away from it all from time to time. He said that if he had been eighteen, he would have liked to live-in because of the social side of it. At the RepGrid encounter, a year after starting the Course, Ben had developed a different perspective on living-in. He had separated from his wife and was now in the nurses home paying ninety pounds a month in addition to his household debts. He reflected on his comments at our first meeting together and added that there was not as much interaction between students as he had expected, but that there was support in the nurses home if required. He found living-in beneficial even if only from the angle of not having to travel into work every day. Previously, he had been driving 28 miles each way to work and eventually college work and shifts had taken their toll. Ben used the room in the nurses home just for sleeping and found it difficult to adapt, but had further involved himself in his outdoor activities which made living-in more tolerable.

Summary

The phenomena of 'living-in, moving-out' or 'living-out, perceptions of living-in' or 'living-out, moving-in' permeated all student accounts in this study. They all had something to say about the effects of accommodation on their being-in-the-world-with-others, whether 'others' were peers or family. The nurses home appears to be an enigma for students entering nursing, but all of them had something to say about it in relation to their development over the period of the Common Foundation Programme. Living-in was seen as an opportunity to develop relationships with the prime objective being support during tough times on the Course, usually related to academic demands. In the early months being in the midst of nursingness had its benefits; offering a cohesive, consistent background to their lives. Toward the end of the Common Foundation Programme, students appeared to need more privacy and space in which they could assert themselves. Primarily they complained of feeling saturated by nursing and stressed their need to socialise with others outside it. This could only be achieved if they moved out of the nurses home and into privately owned accommodation. They still chose to move-in with others in their cohort, although in some relationships, tensions were still running high.

The attention that students paid to the phenomenon of living-in illuminates the importance of being-with-others with similar interests and professional goals. Living-in seemed to provide a necessary bonding opportunity for the young new recruits, although they outgrew the system and required accommodation which continued to give them security and support, alongside independence, freedom of choice and privacy.

173

The student cohort – 'them and us'

This second aspect of 'being-in-the-world-with-others' intends to portray the perceptions of students as they started to identify with certain 'alike' groups of people within their cohort. It became apparent that the notion of 'being against' was more representative of how students were responding to other perceived groups within the cohort. Relationships with others were often strained as a result of age division, perceived irresponsibility toward the Course and often because students felt intimidated in the large group. There are, of course, other examples of 'Them and Us' which could include relationships between students and their patients/clients or supervisors. These relationships are addressed later in this chapter.

The 'mature' students

I am using the term 'mature' to describe those students who were over 26 years old and eligible for an extra allowance with their bursary.

Although there has been some research conducted in nurse education regarding older students (Bond, 1993; Stark and Redding, 1993), there appear to be no empirical studies of older students undertaking nurse preparation programmes alongside younger students, particularly since the introduction of Project 2000 (Glackin and Glackin, 1998).

The three mature students, Ben, Cathy and David, referred to their previous occupations and responsibilities as being valuable in terms of contributing to their current student nurse roles. Ben had a long military history, Cathy had held various public service jobs and David had also had several jobs where he had been in a position to deal with, or relate to, the public. Their main anxieties as they embarked upon the Course focussed on academic work. Despite years of dealing with people, meeting public demands and behaving in a manner acceptable to the public, these mature students were in awe of the standard of written work expected of them. Wheeler and Birtle (1993), believe that older students usually set themselves high standards but bring with them fears and doubts and as a result, develop a poor self concept. The fear of academic failure felt by older students is thought to stem from a greater investment in the Course and therefore having more to lose than younger students. There is also the recognition that this might be their last opportunity to obtain a career. Ben had completed an access course (Whitmarsh, 1993) which he said had prepared him to some extent for the essay writing during the Diploma course. Access courses tend to be part-time, yet in one year students gain the equivalent of two 'A' levels. Cathy had no confidence whatsoever in her abilities to achieve and sustain an academic standard at diploma level, and David, although the most confident of all the students, felt that he would probably need some *polishing up* of his academic skills. These three students all thought that the younger ones were in a more advantageous position, having recently left school or attended other educational institutions for various qualifications.

Ben thought that young students had a fresh outlook on life, while having a lot of living to do. He expected that when these youngsters came across people who needed advice and guidance, in their role as a student nurse, they might struggle. He believed that the younger students might not be able to relate to people as well as a more mature person, but did not hesitate to add that they would be more adaptable in the classroom and better at writing essays. Ben's perceptions of the group as a whole, in the first six months of the Course, were influenced by the segregation of mature students from the younger ones. He felt that there was a barrier between these two age cliques, but claimed that he thought it would be fair to say that it was not formed by the older side of the group. Smithers and Griffin (1986), in their study of higher education students, found that there were amicable relations between older and younger students on the same course, but that the carefree attitude of some younger students, especially towards class participation and attendance, irritated the older students.

Cathy made friends in the group who were slightly younger than herself and joked with me about her being one of the old ones. She had a daughter of sixteen at this stage and told me how she felt she could relate to the younger ones in the group because she could understand them as a result of going through experiences with her daughter. At this early interview, Cathy felt privileged to be given a chance to do nursing. I suggested that working hard had earned her a place on the Course, but she found it difficult to accept that she had as much right to be on it as the younger students. She stated; *I'm lucky coming from nothing - I came out of school with nothing and then being able to do this.* Her personal discipline with coursework can be seen at the various data gathering points - one example is where she told me about her study habits and how she balanced her family and study commitments;

I don't get any disturbances when I go up into where I study, everybody knows, leave me alone. I say how long I'm going to be and I don't go

175

over that. If I say I'm just going to be an hour-and-a-half doing this, then I come down an hour-and-a-half later.

(Cathy, one-to-one interview)

When I first met David he was very busy trying to earn money to support his young family and meet the requirements of the Course through placements and academic study. He worked in a pub in the evenings and in a nursing home at weekends. Lauder and Cuthbertson (1998) question whether older students' problems of finance, childcare and relationship and family responsibilities are faced by men as well as women. David chose to supplement his bursary with part-time employment during the CFP, but gave up some hours when he entered the Branch Programme and encountered different shift patterns. Although his additional work activities may not be representative of all male student nurses it appears to support the belief that being a breadwinner and student can induce financial desperation (Glackin and Glackin, 1998; Kenny, 1998; Lankshear, 1998). David admitted that there was not a minute in any day when he was not doing something. He gave me cause for concern on several occasions when I saw him around the college, as he looked so tired and I wondered how he was coping - juggling his many roles and responsibilities. He told me how he had developed an excellent relationship with his academic tutor who gave him support, and I hoped that he was using the system to his advantage. David appeared confident from the outset and was always frank during discussions with me. He confessed that he had one of the *biggest mouths* in the cohort and that this had got him into trouble occasionally. He was voted student representative, probably he said, because he was vocal. Six months into the Course David believed that the cohort had split into groups and, although he belonged to a small group, he was able to get on with most people. The other students made allowances for him during joint presentations when he had not been able to contribute because of his other responsibilities. At the RepGrid encounter, David was still working one night in the pub and two night shifts in the nursing home. However, he had achieved high marks in his recent assignments which gave him a boost and, although he felt tired, I gathered that he was managing his time effectively. He was concerned that there were students in the cohort who he had never spoken to, but after a year of the Course, the mental health group had found each other and always sat together in lectures. This split had occurred even six months prior to the Branch Programme suggesting that students find a smaller group in which they gain membership because of common interests inside or outside work.

Dreyfus (1991, p6) implies that even when the constituent parts of being-in-the-world try to function as a separate entity they still require the others for their own intelligibility, because they are all constituted through their relationship with the others. He calls this a "normative framework" whereby sense is made of independent things in relation to others. By forming cliques within a larger group students were able to foster appropriate, suitable relationships with others in accordance with age and nursing specialism, for instance. These groups then functioned in isolation to some extent, but drew on the characteristics of the whole cohort to give them a reference for standards, progress and acceptance in nursing and academia.

David expressed how important he thought life experience was to mental health nursing and that bringing up a family was probably of more benefit to the role than spending fifteen years in an office. The frustration experienced by the mature students, that their life experiences were not valued by qualified staff in clinical practice, has been identified by Hufton (1996).

Ben, Cathy and David identified their maturity as a positive attribute whilst learning to be a nurse. They believed that life experience and the lessons learned during the processes involved in raising their families contributed to their ability to relate to patients/clients, but in some ways, isolated them from the rest of the student cohort. This segregation appeared to occur naturally. Students were not divided into groups according to age or specialism by any outside agent. In fact, in my experience, I would say that within college, students are actively separated and re-grouped in order that they have opportunity to discuss issues outside their own peer groups. This is seen to be conducive to developing an open, receptive dialogue between individuals of different backgrounds and interests - an approach required when dealing with the public.

The 'young' students

Seed (1991) found that friendships were initiated and sustained because of the way students were organised in the nurses home and in groups in nursing school. The students in her study were divided according to geographical location of their placements, which she believed impeded contact between individuals in the cohort. This has happened in the past in the area where this research was conducted, where students were allocated to a particular general hospital or community location. As a result, when students came into college they grouped according to geographical location, rather than according to age or nursing specialism as was the case in the present study.

Marie was surprised when a mature student, also in her cohort, was friendly and talkative when they shared a placement. She questioned why this student did not behave in the same way whilst they were in college. Apparently the age groups re-form in college, no matter how well mature and younger students get along on a placement. I think the notion 'united we stand, divided we fall' has some application to this phenomenon; regardless of age, students need support from peers on their placements.

Marie was not bothered about the mature students keeping themselves to themselves, but she complained that they could make more of an effort to socialise. Interestingly she perceived the age divide to be instigated by the mature students, and suggested that the mature students did not have the chance to *stick together* in practice because their placements were randomly allocated. When they returned to college there was opportunity to polarise to their chosen groups again.

I think it's because they've got so much in common. We haven't got children and they have and they have husbands to talk about and they feel that if they're suffering for some reason, they go to talk to someone who can understand a bit more.

(Marie, RepGrid)

Being-with others of a similar age and domestic circumstance appeared to be the most effective support mechanism for students, although mature and young students mixed and provided support for each other at placements when others of a similar age were not available. The basic needs of students appeared to be common in that any of them could provide support for the others because they had a basic universal understanding of one another. Although Heidegger's (p156) object of analysis is individual existence, his analysis also construes sociality as part of the essence of existence. He explains how 'being-with' is always a state of existence for human beings and he claims that even when we are alone, we are being-with but the others are missing. My interpretation of Heidegger's claim is that, though we may be alone physically, we can still be sociable through perceiving, considering and remembering, others.

Similarly, Kelly believes that individuals are in constant interaction with each other and, as a result, each plays a role in relation to others. This is explained through his sociality corollary (Kelly, p66) which enabled me further to interpret the position of mature students within

178

the cohort. He argues that even if people share a common cultural background it does not guarantee social harmony. Each member can misconstrue another's motives and this can be detected in my student data where there is evidence of suspicion of one group towards another. To be able to accept each other and play a constructive role in the social situation, one must not only see eye-to-eye with the person, but also accept their way of seeing things.

Interestingly, Kelly writes;

> One person may understand another better than he is understood. He may understand more of the other's way of looking at things. Moreover, he may understand the other at a higher level of generality. Presumably, if this is true of a certain person with respect to a group of people whose ways of seeing things have some commonality, he is in a strategic position to assume a leadership relation to the group.
>
> (Kelly, 1991, p67)

I considered this in relation to David's position as student representative within the cohort. Did students see him as someone who had sympathy with both 'sides' of the cohort or maybe they actually delegated the job to him to see if it would stem his apparent confidence and verbosity?

The mature student/younger student relationship can also be illuminated through an application of Kelly's commonality corollary (p63). This seems more appropriate in situations where students, regardless of age, develop similar constructions of events not because of their age but because of their stage in the Course.

During their placements students needed each other and related to each other in terms of their development and perceptions of the practical aspects of nursing, even though their experiences may be different. There appears to be a division between mature and younger students on a personal level, but not in the practice context.

Clare told me that she did not have anything in common with the mature students, even though she thought they were *very nice*. A couple of the 'older' students irritated her because she said, *they thought they knew it all*. She accepted that they were likely to have life experience but that she had life experience and that should be valued too. She had been to India for several months back-packing and had learned a great deal about herself and the culture. She thought that knowledge gained through her experience could be as valuable as knowledge gained through experience by a forty-year-old. When she reflected upon these comments, made during the one-to-one interview, Clare recognised that she may have been unfair to the mature students because they made a valuable contribution to discussions in the group. At the RepGrid encounter she had changed her mind about them and was making efforts to get to know a few. Having learned a great deal from the mature students in the group, Clare confessed that her misperceptions of mature students would be a lesson she could take into her staff nurse role.

Carol had similar perceptions of mature students to Clare's. After a year on the Course she had grown to believe that the mature students had similar needs for support as the younger ones. Originally she believed that their lifestyles would not change, but on reflection, she appreciated that they would have to study at home and routines would be disrupted. This realisation affected the way she intended to treat mature students in future.

Sarah claimed that as time progressed students in the cohort polarised to groups in which people *are more like you*. It was interesting to note how Sarah identified people she believed would not complete the Course. Students who had poor attendance at college caused great irritation to those who attended regularly. She said that all students found it difficult to work on placements and go to college and became annoyed when some could not be bothered. Some students in her opinion had very strange ideas about nursing as a career and perceived it to be an easy option. Paula shared Sarah's annoyances and added that some students were so narrow-minded and opinionated that it was difficult to imagine them ever being a nurse. Feeling intimidated by the large group at the beginning, Paula never contributed to discussions. Marie and Clare had similar fears of speaking out in the large group, but all students reported an increase in confidence at the RepGrid encounter when they said that they could contribute to discussions and debates. This took some twelve months to achieve. The younger students felt more able to participate when the cohort was divided into smaller seminar groups. These findings are similar to those of Ashton and Shuldham (1994), who found that small group and seminar work provided support, information and feedback for less vocal students. As a mature student, David noticed how few younger students contributed during discussion sessions. The mature students were always the ones to stimulate discussion and maintain it at the beginning of the Course. Towards the end of the first year, he was pleased that the voices of younger students were eventually being heard. He said it made a change from the usual vocal people in the group.

Summary

'Them and us' was characterised in the group through differences in age and personal interest. There is evidence of some cohesion between different age groups, particularly in clinical practice, where student needs seem to be similar regardless of age, but generally, students divided themselves into age related groups. In addition to being-in-the-world-with-other members of their student group, students also had to learn to be-with their patients/clients and their families.

Being-with patients/clients/relatives - personal investment of Self

"The emotional component of care, like the physical component, is labour in the sense of hard work" (James, 1992, p500), but it has been suggested in the past (Melia, 1984; Seed, 1991) that neophyte nurses must detach from personal contact with patients in order to have the space and energy to develop their ability to perform physical care. White (1996) reported that student nurses had to feel safe to engage in the personal business of their patients and refers to this involvement as "connectedness". I have realised how complex is the development of skills necessary to connect with another as I have trawled through my student participants' data which demonstrates the concept of 'personal investment of Self' in the care of patients and clients. Copp (1997) and James (1992) recognise that the emotional involvement of nurses with their patients/clients is demanding and requires skill. This is evident in the few unique experiences I have selected to portray the phenomenon of 'being-with' patients/clients and relatives apparent in many of the students' stories. I have had difficulty capturing the depth and intensity of relationships and involvement between carers and cared-for. Unlike some other jobs, nursing demands that the carer explores his or her personal attributes in order to examine them in finite detail. It is thought that by doing so the effects that the Self has on others can be identified. The lifeworld of student nurses has been accessed from understandings revealed through reflection. The notion of reflection as a significant factor influencing the development of self-awareness has been recognised by many authors (Boyd and Fayles, 1983; Burns, 1994; Gibbs, 1981; van Manen, 1991). Pierson (1998) makes connections between reflection as it is described in the nursing literature and the work of Heidegger (1966) offering an interesting perspective on reflection as being a prominent component of thought. He does not separate

181

reflection from thought and integrates it with calculative and contemplative thinking; that is, the practical processes involved in thinking, analyses of solutions and instrumental knowledge in contrast to natural and spontaneous processes fundamental to the exploration of meaning. Contemplative thought was evident in the Present Tense Commentaries and Reflective Practice Portfolios and both yielded data rich with evidence of students being-with patients/clients and their relatives. I believe that this occurred as students became aware of the importance of rapport development between nurses and others rather than them focusing their efforts on the practical skills aspect of nursing which was so important to them at the beginning of the Course. 'Being-with', rather than 'doing-to' became central to students' stories as their professional Selves developed. It has been said that being-with is essential if the quality of existence for patients is to be improved (Walters, 1995). [Some of the changes in the nurse's approach to nursing care will be addressed in Chapter 9]. The Present Tense Commentaries and Reflective Practice Portfolios, despite their obvious differences, depended upon the students' skills of reflection in order for them to portray experiences to the listener/reader. Structured reflection was encouraged toward the end of the Course at the time this study was conducted and it is therefore no surprise that experiences of 'being-with' have tended to emerge in the later data collection phases, during the third year of the students' education programme.

In Chapter 7 I was concerned with students' experiences of thrownness and referred to Carol's experience of caring for relatives of a patient [Jim] who had just died. Her reflections upon this incident involving Jim's family are also relevant to this section because she demonstrates her efforts to console them in a personal and professional way. On a personal level she revealed how she imagined it was her father who had died and how she might feel in order to gain a sense of empathy or of really 'being-with'. Throughout her shift she repeatedly returned to the sideroom to give support to Jim's relatives who were waiting for him to die. She panicked when she was left alone with them because she was worried about saying the wrong thing and so adding to the tragedy for them. She was conscious of the effect of her presence on the family and identified a fine line between 'being-there' and being obtrusive. Carol had assumed that as Jim was 'not for resuscitation' the family were aware of his deteriorating condition and were realistically awaiting his death. Despite this she gave them time to talk, cry, say goodbye and begin the separation process. In effect, she had allowed this family to begin to prepare for their loss. She stayed with them, listened and shared her feelings of sadness with them. This personal investment of Self,

182

allowing others to recognise one's own vulnerabilities and showing sadness to people we do not really know can expose the individual and make them vulnerable. Nurses in this type of situation gamble with their own fragility. Professionally, Carol felt that her support was inadequate. Her skills were not well developed or refined enough for her to make more effective decisions which, in her opinion, would have dealt with the relatives more effectively and decreased her vulnerability.

Heidegger refers to the state of 'being towards death' (p295) as ignorance because none of us knows the potential of our own feelings towards it. We may have anxieties or weaknesses which manifest in a number of different ways but we are unable to prepare ourselves for their manifestation. Dasein may cover its own vulnerability by "fleeing in the face" of death (p295). In other words, we make a decision to stay and encounter what might happen, or rescue ourselves from the unknown [as seen in Chapter 7].

I believe that Carol offered her support at regular intervals throughout the day to Jim's relatives because she was aware that to some extent, there was an 'everydayness' to the event. She knew that she would encounter similar situations frequently throughout her career and therefore needed the experience for her professional Self. Heidegger reminds us;

> Death is encountered as a well known event occurring within-the-world. As such, it remains in the inconspicuousness characteristic of what is encountered in an everyday fashion.
>
> (Heidegger, p297)

Pritchard (1995) recognises the stressful nature of dealing with death experiences on an everyday basis, whilst Loftus (1998) highlights the vulnerability of student nurses in such circumstances.

In her Reflective Practice Portfolio Carol stated that she had dealt with numerous bereaved families since this particular incident and had used that experience to help her make decisions. Learning how to act or respond appropriately to individuals whose reaction to death is potentially unpredictable is a very difficult task. It demands an awareness of Self and a knowledge of how one might respond in a situation. Personal awareness may stem from knowledge. For example, Carol used her communication skills with Jim's family and stated that she was aware of their non-verbal cues through body language. She learned in college the importance of communication skills;

I attempted to be aware of their non-verbal signals and also aware of my own which enabled me to sense their need for privacy or for support. My awareness of their non-verbal cues, especially at times of silence, was helpful.

(Carol, Ref. Prac. Port.)

Being-with Jim's relatives meant that Carol shared a deeply emotional and sad time with them. The dying of others is something which Heidegger believes cannot be experienced (p282). I believe it can only be experienced indirectly through the meaning of the incident to those left behind and it is for them that sadness is aroused in me. Being-with bereaved relatives can be traumatic for nurses and requires great skill, but as Heidegger says, "at most, we are always just 'there alongside'" (p282).

Paula's experience of thrownness [see Chapter 7] occurred as a result of being shunned by a patient with whom she had developed a close rapport. Being-with John developed into a 'being-without' as his behaviour toward Paula drove her away from him. She says she stayed away from him for fear of losing her composure. She was confused by her response of reciprocated anger and rejection and questioned whether it occurred because of her own sadness about the diagnosis. Other staff on the ward used avoidance strategies to cope with John's behaviour and their own emotions. Paula recognised, however, that avoidance served to aggravate an already unsatisfactory situation. Paula, like Carol, demonstrated care on a personal level by trying to imagine what it would be like to be told you are terminally ill. She claimed to have gained an understanding of her feelings of sadness and fear and the effects that these had upon her decision making. Being-with those who are dying or have been bereaved demands care derived from both personal and professional Selves. To some extent the care required can be taught and learned, as with communication skills, but many actions depend upon the intuitive nature of the individual. Being-with, in this instance, involves social skills which an individual may or may not have developed. This may be what the mature students alluded to when identifying the possible contribution of maturity at the commencement of the Course - that they have a wealth of experience to bring into testing situations.

The stresses of managing a ward were captured in the reflections written by Cathy during a placement on a five-day surgical ward. She described her concern for an elderly woman [Sara] for whom she had been caring for some time and how Sara's condition had deteriorated whilst Cathy had been organising the transfer of other patients to wards for the weekend. Sara had been a regular admission to the ward and it is apparent from Cathy's description that she had grown fond of her and they had developed a trusting relationship. Cathy became *deeply troubled and sad* that Sara was so ill. Her sense of abandoning Sara played on her mind;

I felt awful about Sara because she was so distressed. During the period of time I spent reassuring her I had given something of myself to her and felt that I had left a job unfinished. These factors affected my decision making.

(Cathy, Ref. Prac. Port.)

During this experience of managing the ward Cathy's role changed from being one of caregiver to manager. She admits to being ill-prepared for this change in role;

I had become emotionally involved with Sara. It would have helped me to discuss my feelings with a qualified member of staff in order to debrief from the role I played in Sara's care to something completely different.

(Cathy, Ref. Prac. Port.)

In this reflective account of her involvement with Sara, Cathy noted that during the course of a shift 'being-with' occurred many, many times and each 'being-with' constituted a different 'being-with' and depended upon the receiver and giver of care.

During a teaching/learning interaction in clinical practice, especially during one-to-one encounters, nurses have sole responsibility for teaching 'good' practice to the patient so that care can be continued at home. Being-with in this type of situation means that nurses must ensure that a 'closeness' is fostered between the nurse and patient so that transfer of knowledge can be effected. In her Reflective Practice Portfolio Marie described a teaching scenario in which she had invested a great deal of herself in terms of effort, knowledge and care, so that a patient she had been nursing should return home with full and accurate information about his diet. 'Being-with' however, does not always result in a rewarding experience for the nurse - in fact 'being-with' many patient/clients can be frustrating, as Marie's reflections revealed. She had cared for a 25 year old man [Tom], in a coronary care unit, who had been admitted with a suspected myocardial infarction [heart attack]. On the day of his discharge from hospital Marie took responsibility for teaching Tom the importance of diet and nutrition if further cardiac problems were to be avoided. She painstakingly prepared her remit with materials to support her teaching from the Health Promotion Department. Her description revealed how she organised the information, assessed Tom's eating habits at home, suggested alternatives for preparing and cooking food and how she had considered making the information interesting. It appeared that despite Marie's efforts, Tom was not happy with many of her suggestions and stated that his girlfriend did the shopping and cooking and he would not like to upset her by suggesting change. Unfortunately, before the teaching session finished Tom was whisked home by his girlfriend who could not stop as a taxi was waiting for them in the car park.

My first impression of Marie's relationship with Tom was that they were possibly operating on several different levels which could include knowledge base, understanding, lifestyle, social class, attitude and self-awareness. These differences constituted an insurmountable obstacle, where Marie functioned on one level and Tom on another due to their contrasting horizons. Marie interpreted this non-fusion of horizons as her failure analysing the teaching session from a very negative perspective. Of course, this may be true, but it is more likely that Tom had no intention of changing his diet. Being-with Tom was never going to be a 'being-with' on a cognitive or emotional level. Being-with Tom meant that Marie would have to accept that Tom had the right to make his own decisions and that she could not take responsibility for him. As a professional, she attempted to give the appropriate, available information. Whether a patient chooses to heed it is their decision and not the nurse's. Understanding 'being-with' patients, clients or relatives incorporates the essence of them as separate individuals who may disagree, react against, disbelieve or choose not to comply with suggestions from professionals. What is important is that, in 'being-with,' individuals show care and concern for one another and realise that others are not the property of Dasein.

Everyday Being-with-one-another maintains itself between the two extremes of positive solicitude - that which leaps in and dominates, and that which leaps forth and liberates.

(Heidegger, p159)

Clare chose to reflect upon a nursing care issue associated with patient advocacy in her portfolio. The reflection centred around her protective, supportive role of a patient with a heroin addiction and how, in her opinion, this patient did not receive appropriate pain relief during an appendicectomy wound dressing change. Clare noticed how some

186

nurses treated this particular person unsympathetically and when she asked why he had not been given analgesia prior to the dressing change the nurse replied "nothing will touch him". Clare thought this lack of analgesia constituted neglect of the patient's needs especially when she witnessed two of his wound dressing changes which caused him so much distress he screamed out loud. On a personal level, Clare reflected upon her own distress during the incident. She felt fear for the patient and angry that he was labelled as 'difficult'. Fearing for the 'other' does not of course, take away his fear - it is simply a 'being-with' during a threatening episode (Heidegger, p181). Clare was apprehensive and anxious about the patient's physical and psychological state and 'fearing for' him was the trigger for her to take further action. From a professional perspective she recognised that she had a responsibility to act as patient advocate. Heidegger describes the implication of 'being-there' as 'understanding' which in turn implies there is some degree of cognition or competence about the situation being experienced. Indeed, 'understanding' is one of Heidegger's central 'existentials' and draws upon the 'ready-to-hand' in order to identify an appropriate solution. Clare had read about Entonox, an odourless gaseous mix of nitrous oxide and oxygen, used as an analgesic for women in childbirth and also at the scene of accidents to provide immediate, virtually harmless, pain relief. Many accident and emergency departments and wards use Entonox for frequent short term relief of pain. Clare considered carefully how Entonox might be appropriate for use with her patient and suggested its use to a senior member of staff. The suggestion was not received graciously with excuses proferred that Entonox was not kept on the ward and special training being required for its administration. The next day however, Clare arrived to start her shift and noticed that the patient had been given Entonox with good effect; the staff nurse had watched a video giving instruction about how to administer it and the cylinder was stored next to the patient's bed. There was no acknowledgement that Clare had suggested the idea, but she felt satisfied that the patient had at last received pain relief.

Clare's experience demonstrated an empathy with her patient, a 'being-with' which meant that she too was distressed when the patient screamed out in pain. Unlike some of her colleagues who were prepared to let this man suffer, apparently as a way of punishing him for his heroin addiction, Clare used her empathy to the advantage of the patient. Reading Clare's reflective episode about the care [or lack of it] given to this patient made me consider the concept of 'being-against' in contrast to 'being-with'. The patient was rendered powerless in the situation - the student had been ignored, and at the outset there was little discussion about the potential of using any analgesia at all. I am reminded that 'being-with' does not necessarily mean 'being-for'. Even though Dasein as 'being-with' lets the Dasein of 'others' be encountered in its world (Heidegger, p157), 'being-with' does not always mean that we matter to, or care for, one another.

Ben disclosed an example of 'being-there' in his Present Tense Commentary. He described the role he played within a paramedic team during an attempted resuscitation of an elderly woman in her home, vividly portraying the environment and the paramedic's actions. The excitement of the full drama was captured, from the moment the call was received at the ambulance station, until the discarded papers and leads were cleared up and disposed of at the end of the resuscitation. The immediacy of the situation of 'being-with' this elderly woman whilst she was unconscious was illuminated by Ben in his description. On arrival at the house, the team ran into the front room;

We are going in there and there's a lady slumped in the chair. I notice that she's very, very grey and also cyanosed. She is very still and her eyes are closed. John goes up and takes her pulse. I don't know why, but I hold her hand.

(Ben, Present Tense Commentary)

Touching has been found to comfort patients and calm them as well as help them to cope (Routasalo and Isola, 1996; Schoenhofer, 1989; Weiss, 1986). Holding a patient's hand provides a sense of identity, reality orientation, reassurance and support and can convey affection and proximity of nurses to their patients (Moore and Gilbert, 1995). This physical gesture of 'being-with' enabled Ben to connect with the woman and obtain a referential context, whereby the meaning of the emergency as a clinical procedure was brought in-line with the sadness of the occasion as witnessed by her daughter, and for the potential ending of a life. Van Manen (1996) sympathises with this type of being-with;

Especially where I meet the other person in his or her weakness, vulnerability or innocence, I experience the undeniable presence of loving responsibility … at the same time I remain sensitive to the uniqueness of the person in this particular situation.

(Van Manen, 1996, p6)

Ben's concern or care for this patient was demonstrated further in his description;

As soon as I stop compressing, the beat on the monitor stops and she's not breathing for herself. The doctor is checking her eyes and there's no reaction to light. He is telling us to stop. I don't really want to, because I've never actually lost one before. But everything is stopping and we are packing everything up. We're cleaning up the area all around and removing all the sharps and pads and the wrappings and different things like that. Then basically we just leave. The last thing I remember of this incident, is looking back at this very small, very frail old lady that up until very shortly before, had been alive ... lying there now in a position that is so undignified. She's lying there with her top cut open and her breasts exposed in a room with the windows wide open onto a main road. I feel so sad and so ... as though I've really let her down, because I've left her in this position. Not because I've failed to save her; she died, that was natural ... but because we haven't covered her up and we haven't made her decent.

(Ben, Present Tense Commentary)

This Present Tense Commentary portrays Ben's personal need to finish the caring for this elderly woman by covering her up at the end of the resuscitation attempt and by making her presentable for her relatives. He described how his professional duties were in conflict with his personal values and how he had felt a strange *sense of connection and shared struggle* with the woman. This shared struggle was Ben's 'being-with' this woman. Even in an event such as this, where the 'other' was unconscious it is apparent that Dasein can still make a connection with the 'other'. It is an empathy for, concern for, shared struggle with, the 'other'. Ben also used the term 'being there' to describe his helping role within the team which he claimed helped to offset the negative feelings which gave him a sense of incompleteness and not finishing the job. Ben's Present Tense Commentary gave me especial insight into the meaning the events had for him. The technique was particularly useful in enabling students to reflect and recall situations where they thought their caring was not apparent. By reliving the experience, Ben certainly facilitated his own process of self-forgiveness for his regrets during the incident with the elderly woman. The event was so significant to him that he also chose to use it as one of the episodes in his Reflective Practice Portfolio.

David, in his Present Tense Commentary, described how he attempted to 'be-with' a woman in a mental health setting who appeared confused and distressed because she could not remember that her husband had died, and she wanted to meet with him. She became upset and agitated when nursing auxiliaries repeatedly told her that he had been dead for fifteen years, with little regard for the woman's feelings or understanding of the situation. David intervened and in order to achieve 'being-with' this client on a similar psychological dimension, used reminiscence to help her to recall and recognise that her husband was no longer alive. He talked me through this process;

The first thing I say to her is er 'Do you always see your husband at this time of day?' She says 'yes'. I then lapse into the past tense and say 'It must have been nice, chatting to your husband at this time of the day, what did you do with him?'. Although that is taking her mind off it, it's also enabling her to talk about her husband. The upshot of it all is that she is able to talk about her husband and recognise the fact that he has passed away; but it isn't a hurtful feeling for her because she was able to remember the good times with him as well. I am able to utilise the skills that I've got in reflection and also in reminiscence, but without upsetting her that the fact is that her husband did die fifteen years ago and this made me feel really good and she is happy and I'm happy at the end of this, and the aim has been achieved.

(David, Present Tense Commentary)

David recognised that the strategies used by the nursing auxiliaries were ineffective. He assessed the situation and created a therapeutic interaction whereby his understanding of the client's distress enabled him to 'be-with' her and connect with her in her moment of psychological turmoil. David also demonstrated his desire to empathise with a young man he was caring for who had been admitted with suicidal tendencies. In order to plan care for this client, David believed that he must try to imagine how life could be so bad that his client was prepared to take his own life. David wrote;

I realise on reflection of this scenario, that my complete, unadulterated joy for living made it extremely difficult for me to empathise with someone wanting to kill themself. I tried to imagine the worst possible scenario for myself. My wife and children are all killed on the same day that my house is repossessed and I fail this assignment. Yet, I still could not find myself able to come up with an emotion that was severe enough for me to want to commit suicide.

(David, Ref. Prac. Port.)

In his analysis, David explored his own feelings associated with this particular client and came to the realisation that instead of trying to create disturbance within himself to empathise with clients a more

190

effective strategy would be to simply accept that there were people with suicidal tendencies. Simply using this non-judgmental acceptance allowed him to work more closely with this client group rather than struggle to 'be-with' them on a more empathic level. Knowing oneself, Heidegger claims (p161), is grounded in being-with. Understanding is developed through an acquaintance with others and disclosure of Self to 'others'. Apparently, knowing oneself can be lost in aloofness - an attempt to hide oneself away or to put on a disguise rather than opening oneself up to others (Heidegger, p161). Heidegger also states that it is problematic to try to understand the 'psychical life of others'. In mental health settings, nurses are required to do just that and David's personal and professional development is apparent in these examples of 'being-with' his clients, although the intensity of relationships in mental health settings means that development might occur in students only if they are closely supervised (Bodley, 1991; Hartman, 1984).

In being-with, caring and caring presence are evident. It is thought that to presence oneself (Benner, 1984) with another means that one is available to understand and be-with another (Nelms, 1996). Benner (1984) referred to presencing as situating the nurse's self 'sensitively' and 'imaginatively' in the world of those being cared for. I would argue that it takes a substantial amount of experience to know how to 'sensitively' and 'imaginatively' presence oneself in the world of others, and this may be another reason why students did not talk, to any great extent, about rapport with patients/clients before their late second/third year.

Summary

In this section I have attempted to convey the intensity of relationships between patients/clients/relatives and nurses through the concept of 'being-with'. It appears that a connectedness can be achieved between people on a personal, professional, physical and subconscious level. The students explored their practice using reflection-on-action, as described by Schon (1983), and have captured the essence of experience in the Present Tense Commentaries and Reflective Practice Portfolios. I complete this section with a quote from Sarah which I consider summarises the challenge and delight of 'being-with' people;

I think it's when I go out and I'm with someone ... like if it's an old woman and I'm doing her leg ulcer (dressing), or something like that and afterwards she says 'thanks love' ... it's like if someone's in the bed and they're uncomfortable and you can do something about it and make them feel comfortable again and there's a smile on their face when they go to sleep. You just can't beat that feeling. I get a real buzz out of it. Whatever it is, it can be just feeding somebody or giving a commode, it doesn't matter. It's important for that person and when I've finished whatever I'm doing and I walk away, I know I've helped in some way. You can't beat that. What job beats that? I don't think there is one.

(Sarah, RepGrid)

Experiences of learning in clinical practice: being-with supervisors

The influence of qualified nurses and supervisors on Project 2000 student nurses development in the clinical area has been identified in the work of Burdett (1998), MacLeod Clark, Maben and Jones (1996), White, Riley, Davies and Twinn (1993) and Wilson-Barnett, Butterworth, White, Twinn, Davies and Riley (1995). Various definitions of supervision are proposed in the nursing literature (Catmur, 1995; Ford and Jones, 1987; Rolfe, 1990), and the term is used interchangeably with 'preceptor', 'mentor', 'assessor' and 'tutor' (Castledine, 1994). In my work area student nurses were assigned to a particular qualified nurse at each placement, who was responsible for enabling the student to realise their learning objectives and for negotiating appropriate clinical experience with the student. This person, the 'supervisor', had an obligation to ensure that they met with 'their' students at regular intervals and had a knowledge of the Course and likely needs of the student. They were expected to disseminate specialist skills and knowledge pertaining to the area in which they worked. From my study it was particularly noticeable that these specific individuals acted as role models to the fledgling nurses more toward the end of the Course, when the attitudes, skills and approach to managing the job of nursing became a focus for students' attentions. In contrast, Holloway's study in 1995, revealed that students required less supervisory structure to their practice as 'trainees' progressed through 'levels of practice experience'. My study suggested however, that students took note of the ways their supervisors used professional skills to manage their human, equipment and financial resources. Students in MacLeod Clark et al.'s study (1996) contributed to a list of characteristics which they believed constituted a good nursing role model. Interpersonal skills, nursing knowledge, caring, professional

192

skills, personal qualities, openness to the potential for change and organisational and management skills were listed as key features (p96). However, there is evidence to suggest that problems have been identified surrounding the supervisory role and contact with supervisors, as experienced by Project 2000 students (White et al., 1993).

Several studies (Bradby, 1990; Hughes, 1985; Olsson and Gullberg, 1987; Shead, 1991) have identified the importance of students receiving support from clinical staff and some see this as part of a normative process, whereby the neophyte moves closer to the expectations of the professional group.

Feeling well supported, trusted and having a good role model are identified in Carol's reflections upon her first attempt at managing a ward during a third year placement. She described how her supervisor had prepared the environment for her, so that the staff knew that Carol was 'in charge' and could contribute to her feeling of being supported.

From my perspective I felt that I was trusted which, due to my student status and previous minimal experience within management, made me feel quite privileged.

(Carol, Ref. Prac. Port.)

From this statement, one could assume that students did not always receive the support they required to learn on-the-job. Feeling privileged because one is receiving adequate supervision implies that this episode is the exception rather than the rule.

Carol had observed her supervisor on previous shifts operating a democratic leadership style and noticed how she engaged in discussion with other staff before making decisions. This set the scene for a positive experience for Carol which, in turn, enabled her to manage human resources and time effectively and fostered an appreciation for the effects on the person managing the ward, of a good staffing ratio and appropriate skill mix.

Paula identified one particular occasion where she had been poorly supervised in practice and characterised this as the supervisor having little time for her, so that her learning needs were not identified, let alone met. Paula claimed that her supervisor used an autocratic supervisory style and rather than discussing issues about practice, allocated tasks to her which became repetitious so that she felt her learning was minimised. As a consequence, there was little opportunity to be self-directed and this, combined with negative emotions, resulted in Paula confronting her supervisor which in turn led to the supervisor becoming hostile toward her.

She stated that I was in no position of power to criticise and reinforced that she was too busy.

(Paula, Ref. Prac. Port.)

Feeling respected and working as equals were identified by Paula as important in learning how to function in a team. Whilst acknowledging that the supervisor had experience, the need for mutual respect and a de-structuring of the traditional nursing hierarchy might have contributed toward a more open, productive relationship between student and supervisor. In my experience, mutual respect is rewarded by admiration, and students who are treated in a dignified manner by their supervisors earn their allegiance, with the placement often gaining the reputation of a good learning environment. Interestingly, Paula's bad experience of supervision occurred in an accident and emergency department which she said conjured up a picture of danger, unstable emotions and highly charged situations, which her experience of supervision in the department consolidated. Paula recognised that inevitably this knock to her own self-esteem and confidence would have an effect on the care she gave to patients. She also added that it took some time to regain her confidence on successive placements.

Ben also described an experience of what he called an autocratic supervisory style. Like Paula, he felt the management system on the ward was too strict, resulting in him feeling *oppressed*. His uncomfortable experience of supervision arose as a result of qualified staff feeling betrayed by managers in practice. Ben comments that there was *undischarged hostility* amongst supervisors, which in turn affected students who were seen to be another source of stress and anxiety in an already volatile social environment. Situations where there is tension within staff groups have been identified as a common source of stress for students (Scully, 1980).

Within my study there is evidence to suggest that some risk is involved when the supervisor adopts a parenting role. Treating students like children, such as delegating tasks without rationale and over-protection, leads to a dependence and decline of existing abilities in students. Paula identified in her reflections that the supervisor may have tried to preserve her own role against somebody whom she perceived to be threatening. Allocating tasks and occupying the student with trivial activities meant that she had less chance of being asked testing questions. It transpired through Paula's reflections that this particular supervisor had no previous experience of supervising students. She felt confused about the expectations of the role and may well have felt unsupported herself.

194

For Carol, having an experienced supervisor, who was obviously clear about the demands of the role, meant that she was able to work autonomously but with support. She discussed her performance after her ward management attempt with her supervisor and this enabled Carol to reflect on the opportunity and identify strengths and limitations.

White et al. (1993) found that without exception, the process of assessing students in mental health nursing practice actively involved discussion and students' self-assessment. Subsequently, supervisors made a second set of judgements, and discrepancies between scores were discussed and reconciled. However, there were many problems identified with assessment in practice, including the student not working consistently with one person, the subjectivity of the whole process and supervisors not being skilled in the use of documentation. Similarly, Green (1994) argued that if student-centred learning methods are being advocated there is a clear indication that self-assessment should be introduced into assessment procedures. In Paula's experience, discussion did not take place and the supervisor made judgements about her performance which were perceived by Paula to be misinformed.

Heidegger (p83) believes that being-with is about concern - "looking after it, considering, attending to something". Leaving undone, neglecting and renouncing he says, are also ways of concern but in a "deficient mode" in which the possibilities of concern are kept to a bare minimum. My understanding of students not receiving appropriate supervision in clinical practice may be viewed in Heidegger's terms as a form of neglect. But I believe that this neglect is not a malicious attempt to disable the student; rather, it occurs as a result of the competing demands upon the supervisors in their multiple roles within the clinical environment. It could be argued, the majority of clinical staff operate in the 'deficient mode' as a strategy for self-preservation in a climate of staff shortages and demand upon their time. This results in supervisors having to prioritise requests for attention so that students' learning needs do not always take precedence.

Within her Present Tense Commentaries, Cathy described both good and inadequate supervision experiences. Having arrived on a ward for her first shift, Cathy looked for an advocate and some guidance in processes and routines on the new ward. She was given the report from the night shift and described the tension created by not being able to identify people or their position in the hierarchy because none of them wore name badges;

I don't know who is an auxiliary and who's a staff nurse and who's the sister. So, I'm trying to make sense of everything and looking at the

195

board for information on the ward layout and even the doctors' names
are unfamiliar - so I'm just trying to make sense of that.

(Cathy, Present Tense Commentary)

Her dismay within this new environment was apparent until the sister allocated her to a staff nurse with whom she was supposed to work during the shift. However, the staff nurse disappeared for the rest of the morning and Cathy was left to fend for herself. Cathy had intended to shadow the staff nurse and observe how she prioritised her day. The supervisor thought that the student should be capable of continuing with the usual routine of the morning and give basic care to her allocated patients. This is an undesirable outcome for the student, the supervisor and certainly for patients. On reflection, Cathy commented that this scenario could have been avoided if she had been more assertive and insisted on supervision, or if she had made plans to visit the ward informally, meet with her supervisor and agree how they should work together.

It was ridiculous how the whole thing panned out. Perhaps I was feeling
under the weather myself. But as I say, a ward placement is so different
to being on the community and everybody seems to be rushing around.
The staff nurse I was with, she was very busy; that sort of rushing around
type of person and that didn't help me. It just really made me more
anxious.

(Cathy, Present Tense Commentary)

Anxiety and a sense of isolation are common responses to being in an unfamiliar environment without supervision (Hyland, Millard and Parker, 1988). Being-without-others could be interpreted as neglect, as previously stated, but may simply result from misunderstandings or the supervisor misconstruing the situation. The supervisor judged Cathy's abilities on her length of time on the Course. This approach to supervision is common amongst those supervisors who have been used to the traditional style of training [normative socialisation] where all students had the same types of placement at the same time, resulting in similar experiences and an almost standard progression through the Course (Spouse, 1996). With the Diploma programme in existence at the time of this study students were allocated to different placements at different times in the Course thereby gaining different experiences in their first, second and third years. The damage which can be caused to individual student's development through labelling them according to stage of the Course cannot be overestimated. In contrast with the first episode, Cathy ran her second commentary based upon a good experience with a supervisor whilst she was in the community with a health visitor. The scenario was very different and Cathy demonstrated how efficiently the health visitor communicated with her and how they planned their working day together. The health visitor's respect for the student is evident in Cathy's commentary –

I'm walking into the playgroup and my health visitor introduces me as her colleague. This makes me feel equal to her, rather than somebody who is a student and um perhaps wouldn't give as good a service as a colleague would.

(Cathy, Present Tense Commentary)

It's about being valued. And another thing was, I was just encouraged all the time and it was very definite what I was going to do and we had talked about it and the preparation was there.

(Cathy, Present Tense Commentary)

Cathy found the one-to-one supervision enabled her to develop skills and confidence. The staff nurse in the 'inadequate supervision' scenario made her feel anxious because she was always rushing around and appeared not to have time for her. The health visitor, on the other hand, for what ever reason, was able to give undivided attention and also made time for feedback and discussion.

The vulnerability of students in clinical practice is illuminated by Marie in her commentary; she chose a situation where she felt bullied by a qualified counterpart. Marie arrived on a new placement where everyone was rushing around, knowing what they were doing; no-one welcomed her or suggested that she work with another member of staff. She commented *I think I'll just stand here for another five minutes and then I better go and do something.* After this time had elapsed, Marie decided to ask the staff nurse if she would like her to wash and dress a patient. The staff nurse answered "yes" without any other explanation. After several minutes, whilst Marie and a fellow student had taken it upon themselves to wash one of the female patients, the staff nurse came over to them and shouted "Leave the bed - leave everything - just put the patient in the chair" and then walked off. In reliving this experience Marie herself shouted loudly to imitate the way the staff nurse had spoken to them. The volume startled me as generally students had been quietly spoken during their commentaries. The episode had affected her deeply and she really wanted me to understand how she had been made to feel by the staff nurse. Sartre (1996, p414) explains how

197

'being-for-others' precedes 'being-with-others' because one has to have an understanding of the 'others' perspective before they can become 'we'. When this does not occur in an interaction conflict arises. After Marie's commentary I asked how she dealt with the situation and she replied;

I avoided her and luckily she went home. When I went back the next day she wasn't there ... I thought, I'm not going to like this and I've got two months of her.

(Marie, Present Tense Commentary)

On reflection she added;

I definitely wouldn't speak to people like that now, never mind when I'm a staff nurse. But I mean, no way would I speak to a student like that. I probably looked terrified anyway, the first day ... you just don't talk to people like that, it's bad manners.

(Marie, Present Tense Commentary)

Taking advantage of students in their already powerless position has been a theme in my students' accounts. They talk of their experiences in practice where they were used for mundane jobs such as taking or collecting equipment or patients to and from other wards or departments. Because they appeared to be additions to the established team, other nurses exploited their supernumerary position.

Clare reflected upon an experience she had on the first day of her rostered service placement which, she explained, had implications for delegation, supervision and support in clinical practice. A senior nurse asked Clare's supervisor if she could 'borrow' her to escort a patient to the X-ray department. The senior nurse pressured Clare's supervisor who eventually agreed to Clare going. I think it is important that the reader has full exposure to the way that Clare told her story in her Reflective Practice Portfolio, rather than using my own words:-

They [the supervisor and senior staff nurse] *took me to the patient who was in pain and receiving oxygen. She looked quite ill. I knew nothing about the patient, her diagnosis or the reason for the X-ray and nothing was explained to me. I stated that I was not sure if I should take the patient because the X-ray department was a long way away and I was inexperienced. She played down my concerns and they were not taken on board. When we got to the X-ray department we had to wait a long time and the patient began to complain of pain in her chest. I reassured her and made her as comfortable as possible and asked a passing member of staff how much longer we would have to wait. The pain got worse while the patient was having her X-ray. I spoke to a porter expressing my concerns that we get the patient back to the ward as quickly as possible. On the way back the patient was in considerable pain. When we arrived back the staff nurses took over. Lots of nurses and doctors were bustling around the patient. When I went to see the patient I was asked to go and help in another bay. Within two hours of arriving back on the ward, the patient had died. I was not told this directly. I knew instinctively but when I asked they told me simply to look behind the curtains. This was my first experience of death of a patient. I attempted to discuss my feelings with the staff, but they appeared too busy.*

(Clare, Ref. Prac. Port.)

This account demonstrates neglect of the student's needs and furthermore how patients are endangered because of staff shortages. Clare described how anxious she felt during the whole episode and stated that when she was told to look behind the curtains, she felt shocked, frightened, confused, sad and bewildered because only two hours previously she had been having a conversation with this woman. Having this task delegated to her by the senior staff nurse and her supervisor, who incidentally should have protected both the patient and the student, made Clare feel responsible for the patient's death. Clare was in a position of powerlessness and felt intimidated and vulnerable - indeed she said that she feared disapproval and rejection by her supervisor which could have affected the outcome of the placement for her. Indeed, Being-with supervisors caused students anxiety because of the subjectivity of assessment of practice. Assessment of performance in practice has been criticised for this (Jarvis, 1983; Price, 1986; While, 1991; Wong and Wong, 1987; Wood 1982) and in some instances students have been judged before they have even had a chance to demonstrate development of skills (While, 1992; Wood, 1982). Students in White et al.'s study (1993) also commented on the subjectivity of the whole assessment process and recognised the influence that other factors could have on the process, particularly relationships between supervisor and student.

Establishing a relationship with her supervisor whilst out with the paramedics meant that Sarah developed a work routine in which she felt valued and was able to contribute to the team. One individual particularly encouraged Sarah to perform tasks under supervision and boosted her confidence through positive feedback which Hawkins and

Shohet (1989) acknowledge is an important aspect of the supervisory role. On one occasion she attended an emergency where she was unable to participate because the team of paramedics were not the usual she went out with. She felt so inadequate that the intensity of the situation and her inability to participate reduced her to tears. She talked this over with her paramedic supervisor who reassured her and commented that she was a capable student and that it was just one incident where she perceived that she had not performed appropriately. The incident also provides some evidence for the importance of consistency in supervision (Berragan, 1997; White et al. 1993). Sarah concluded;

It was just that the ambulance men I was out with ... they were both great guys, but they weren't the ones I was used to ... I didn't have the rapport with them, that I had with the others.

(Sarah, Present Tense Commentary)

Sarah also commented in her Reflective Practice Portfolio that on occasions in practice she had no supervision at all. These inconsistencies of standard and the amount of supervision meant that students had to gauge each new placement and decide how to achieve their learning outcomes and what their strategy could be, depending upon the mood, ability, flexibility and commitment of the assigned supervisor. Those who were in a position of student advocate frequently ignored the learning needs of students and became their opponents causing insecurity and problems with settling into placements.

Summary

In this chapter, I have presented examples of the students' experiences in relation to 'Living in - moving out', 'Them and us - the student group', 'Being-with patients/clients and relatives and personal investment of Self' and 'Learning in clinical practice - being-with supervisors'. These experiences illuminated the concept 'being-in-the-world-with-others' and, although they may not represent any other student population, many might recognise similarities with their own experiences.

It is through encounter and interaction with others that these experiences arose. Through being-with-others the students learned to tolerate, consider, enjoy, understand and sojourn with people as part of a transient population who take on a nomadic type of existence for three years both in their personal and professional lives. They realised that an acquaintance with Self occurs through the interaction with others as Heidegger (p161) informs us, "Knowing oneself is grounded in being-with". These encounters occurred in the nurses accommodation where students enjoyed the camaraderie and support during the early months of the Course and then felt the need to move out because of lack of privacy and intensity of focus upon nursing. Interactions, or lack of them, became apparent when mature and young students divided into factions within the cohort which caused some tension within the group in college, but some solidarity was developed between students of different ages in clinical practice. Being-with patients/clients, their families and supervisors showed how students invested their energies in caring relationships and how misunderstandings between students and their supervisors resulted in students' needs not being met in the clinical environment.

In the next chapter, Heidegger's concept of 'temporality' is used as a framework to describe and explain some of the students' development during the Diploma of Higher Education in Nursing Studies course. In the main, the chapter addresses the theme which dominated the students' accounts; Being a student - Being a nurse.

9 Temporality - Being a Student, Being a Nurse

Time provides the ultimate bond in all relationships.

(Kelly, p58)

In Chapter 8 four distinct areas of being-in-the-world-with-others were identified from students' accounts. Examples from the students' data illuminated being-with their student counterparts in the nurses' home; amongst others in the student cohort; giving of themselves to patients/clients/relatives, and also in relationships with supervisors in clinical practice. Caring and caring presence were identified as key features in interactions with others and the essence of Dasein was captured as being-with on an everyday basis.

As the purpose of the Diploma of Higher Education in Nursing Studies course is to transform students into professional nurses it is important that experiences which contribute to that development are examined. In this chapter I aim to demonstrate changes in my participants' constructs as a result of processes, development, movement and transformation over time. Much of the material for this chapter was gathered in the original one-to-one interviews which gave a baseline of experience, and then subsequently in the RepGrid encounters, Present Tense Commentaries and Reflective Practice Portfolios, where students demonstrated their changing perceptions and behaviours.

I have endeavoured to appreciate the students' stories as manifestations of a distinct separate reality with a logic, a consistency and an integrity all of their own. I also acknowledge through this chapter that participants are not static, but that their constructions of events reflect the past, present and future of their experience.

In Chapter 6, I showed how students had comportment toward the Course and nursing, which can be seen as the arrival stage on a journey through a multitude of reconstructions. How they construed the Course and nursing at the beginning of their nurse education programme, provided me with an understanding of their naïve, untainted perceptions of what was to come. As a result of six months experience on the Course and at placements students' constructs changed, often accompanied by disappointment, sometimes by regret, but mostly with acceptance. This 'past' resembles past values about nursing, caring and personal values of Self in relation to the job of nursing. Indeed, Heidegger (p20) states that the aim of any individual is the interpretation of time as a possible horizon for any understanding of 'being'.

'Being a student' and 'being a nurse' were two polarised aspects of students' accounts and it is my intention to explore these aspects and then present some of my interpretations within a hermeneutic and personal construct theory framework.

A major distinction between the CFP and Branch Programmes

For the participants in my study, the CFP was seen as the 'student' part of the Course despite the numerous placements that they attended. This initial eighteen months represented various aspects of nursing, so that students gained an insight into the multidimensional role of the nurse and an understanding of the needs of society in relation to health. The Common Foundation Programme was perceived by students to be a time of testing their stamina to survive the Course, an initiation where the individual endured the agonies of academic work and placements, which were reported to be of little interest, in order to access the 'real' part of the Course - the Branch Programme. Once students moved into the Branch Programme their motivation increased, they were more able to apply theory to practice and they had a mission to complete. Participants saw the CFP as emphasising the 'student' role while the Branch Programme enabled individuals to access the 'nurse' role. But there were varying degrees of the role in both the CFP and the Branch Programme, and this is where the two roles appeared to conflict.

Contrary to what I have argued elsewhere, that students do not undergo a standard development process, there appears to be a significant shift in all students' perceptions of the Course between the CFP and Branch Programmes. This is a common characteristic in all students' narratives which may occur because of the content and organisation of the Course.

Academic work in the CFP

In their stories of being a student, participants conveyed their anxieties about assignments, college expectations, problems with the student role and the panic which resulted from their perception that they were not learning practical skills.

Their construct of the 'student' part of their role was dominated by the unexpected demands of a Diploma course. Despite being prepared for more theory than she had envisaged on a traditional nursing course, Marie commented upon the amount of reading expected of students and how the content of the curriculum had little application to what she was seeing and doing on placements. There is evidence to suggest that she made no link between sociology, psychology and the role of the qualified nurse. In their first interviews students perceived the nurse as a skilled, practical individual and their desire to learn was firmly rooted in the ability to perform tasks rather than to acquire and utilise knowledge. To be a nurse was to master tasks. Ben stated that *being a student you know nothing, being a nurse means that you can do something practical.*

Through the student grapevine students quickly took on board which were the 'difficult' semesters. Getting through these semesters was seen as a milestone and students often saw this as reaching a goal which motivated them to achieve the next goal - another semester, another assignment. This way of construing the Course appears to be short-sighted in that short-term goals are met, but cause the student to perceive the Course composed of many small chunks rather than as a continuous learning experience. Linking experiences and transferring skills and knowledge from one situation to another is hindered through this short term goal approach.

In my study anxieties about academic work were equally intense in the younger and mature students and their reasons for anxiety were similar. Mature students' perceptions that younger students might perform better academically, because of their recent exposure to essay writing for instance, were refuted by the experiences of Marie and Sarah who both had recently studied at diploma and degree levels and were as anxious as their older counterparts.

Inherent in the role of being a student was the apparent onset of panic and anxiety associated with academic assignments and the distress experienced at results time. Part of this anxiety originated from a guessing game motivated by the question, 'who are the markers and what exactly are they looking for?' During the initial interview, Ben disclosed that he had already re-written his Anatomy and Physiology (A&P) assignment because he was convinced that he had been referred. He was awarded a mark of 80% and I asked him how his perception of his work could be so out of synchrony with the markers. He retorted that students get different ideas about what is wanted by tutors and gave an example

204

of a student who had given an identical piece of work to two tutors. He said that one gave feedback that the work was *garbage* and the other wanted it to be used as a good example for future students *it's pot luck whether you get a sociology teacher or a health studies teacher marking an assignment* (RepGrid).

The feeling that the Course appeared too theoretical was shared by most of the participants in this study - Ben's comment *we want to be nurses not sociologists* (RepGrid) represented the perception that nursing studies appeared to be secondary to theoretical components within the CFP. Like Ben, Sarah thought that she had done badly in the A&P assignment. It transpired that she, too, had done well (74%). Despite her previous essay writing experience, Sarah found it difficult to come to terms with the amount and standard of work required. Throughout the CFP she continually questioned her ability to succeed, which prevented her from enjoying aspects of the Course. Sarah also talked of her *disorientation* related to the role of the nurse and how learning theory in college and then skills in practice felt disconnected during the early months. She considered that if she was having difficulties, it would be really terrifying for those who had no academic preparation.

Despite his responsibilities, David fared well in his assignments but admitted that they were always rushed. Like Ben and Sarah, David was unsure whether he had satisfied the requirements because of conflicting advice and misinterpretations of the guidelines. At the beginning of the Course he stated that theory and practice were disjointed and that the balance did not seem right.

These stories coincide with findings from studies by House (1975) and Luker (1984), who identified the dilemma graduate nurses faced when there was conflict between the skills developed at university and those required for work; the intellectual and social skills developed in the academic environment compared with practical skills demanded in the workplace. The CFP appeared to assist the socialisation of student nurses into the student role rather than the desired nurse role, with its perceived emphasis upon the academic requirements of the Course rather than on students learning practical skills and going to the desired institutional placements.

Building up a total picture of the nurse's role and how to achieve this through the Course occurred slowly and old constructs were not necessarily precursors to new ones. Being a nursing auxiliary for example often had less mileage in terms of benefit than originally perceived, yet gaining insight into the role had other advantages not previously envisaged. This fragmentation of experience demonstrates what Kelly (p59) refers to as "a stream of consciousness whose headwaters, terrain and flood potential may result in the cutting out of new channels or the erosion of old ones". The value of this type of experience is that individuals are able to distinguish between alike and different events, thus expanding the range of convenience of their constructs. Inconsistencies within constructs may be reconciled through various means; reinterpreting the event so that it can be assimilated or by altering an opinion one holds of oneself for example. Similar constructs held by another individual may not be fragmented at all. Davis (1975) proposed a socialisation framework which identified 'labelled recognition of incongruity' as his second stage. This appears to capture the essence of the fragmentation corollary whereby students, after receiving feedback from teachers, realised that their expectations did not correspond to the college's expectations. Participants in my study said that they often felt in competition with each other rather than working together, like Davis' students, to find a solution. Students admitted to feeling isolated because of their contrasting styles of learning and varying abilities to keep pace. Davis' framework provides a useful staged analysis of the lived experience of students in the 1970s. It is not however, an all-encompassing model for students undertaking Project 2000 courses.

An overview of students' constructs regarding academic work can be seen in Table 9.1. Four profiles can be identified. David was the only student to perceive himself as having academic confidence and an ability to apply theory to practice during the late stages of the CFP. I have called this a 'consistent' positive profile.

Carol, Clare, Marie and Sarah, unlike David, were not confident and did not have the ability to apply theory to practice, even during the late stages of the CFP. I have called this a 'consistent' negative profile.

There are three students with inconsistent profiles. Although she had academic confidence, Paula was not able to make a connection between theory and practice while Ben and Cathy were not confident in their academic work, they could apply theory to practice.

It is interesting to note at this stage that there appears to be no difference in academic performance between male and female students although four of the five 'young' students were consistently negative in academic profile. I also find it interesting that the only student who had studied at degree level was one of two who had an assignment referred.

206

CFP

	Academic experience Pre-course	Academic Confidence	Application of Theory to Practice (late stage of CFP)	Assignment Results
David	'A' Level	Yes	Yes	7 Pass
Paula	GCSE	Yes	No	7 Pass
Ben	Access course	No	Yes	7 Pass
Cathy	'O' Level	No	Yes	7 Pass
Carol	GCSE	No	No	6 Pass, 1 Refer
Clare	'A' Level	No	No	7 Pass
Marie	Diploma / B.Tec	No	No	7 Pass
Sarah	Degree	No	No	6 Pass, 1 Refer

Academic work in the Branch Programmes

In the early stages of the Branch Programmes all students began to reconstrue theoretical aspects of the Course and some had made links between theory and practice. At this time they were experiencing placements in clinical areas associated with their chosen branch of either adult general or mental health nursing. Marie commented that the theory side of the Course was much clearer to her and showed assimilation of theory to her practice. Unlike other participants in this study, Marie enjoyed the theoretical input more than the practical side toward the end of the Course. She viewed the opportunity to study at home as a period of remission from practice, where she had a break from the physical demands of nursing. Marie learned from Course tutors that she could not be expected to read all the suggested literature and so concentrated on essential texts and articles which enabled her to write the assignments with less anxiety.

The frustrations and confusions for Ben arose from an inability to perceive how theory was useful to practice during the early stages of the CFP but in his Reflective Practice Portfolio he described a gradual change in his construing of the usefulness of theory to practice. This realisation occurred because he could make a contribution to discussions about nursing practice and, in return, his contribution was valued by the nursing team. Having a knowledge base also enabled him to make decisions about practice which previously had been made by other, more senior, members of the team. This increased his self-esteem which led to a desire to gain more knowledge.

Sarah revisited her comments about not knowing what tutors wanted in assignments and claimed that she 'misjudged' the requirements in the past. Reflecting on her struggle with the academic aspects of the Course, she admitted that if the guidelines were followed and the student handbook consulted then it would be likely a student would pass. Sarah's portrayal of the panic experienced en masse by students seven weeks before an assignment submission date illustrates a common experience for all students. At the RepGrid encounter in the CFP she had talked about how her confidence with the academic side of the Course ebbed and flowed. During the Branch Programme she adopted a much more positive outlook and stated that she hoped to go on to do a degree. She talked about 'piecing the bits together' and rationalised the need for academic study in nursing in terms of nurses needing knowledge to function.

Sarah's recognition that learning should occur throughout her nursing career developed as a result of understanding priorities. She described how she coped with adapting to two very different roles when she was working in the community. On this particular occasion, Sarah had been with a young woman who was terminally ill and described how she had been talking to her for two hours whilst out with the district nurse. She then had to rush off to Pizzaland to fulfil her role as waitress in her part time job. It was evident that she found the transition sufficiently difficult that it often resulted in her being intolerant as a waitress. She had also started to value learning experiences in college and enjoyed lively debates with her peers which resulted in her appreciation of others' viewpoints.

Clare managed to change her study habits at the onset of the Branch Programme, having realised that she spent a lot of her time and energy worrying about assignments. She reflected that the experience had taught her to cope with pressure and refine her time management skills. The feeling of being overwhelmed by theory had decreased dramatically by the Branch Programme and Clare talked about settling down to a pace and setting priorities in terms of workload.

Paula had also started to develop academic confidence at this stage and had realised that there was no one to 'give her a push' as in general education. She had developed an appreciation of the importance of theory and was also beginning to make links to practice.

An overview of students' constructs regarding academic work in the Branch Programmes can be seen in Table 9.2.

Table 9.2 shows how six of the eight students developed a profile in which they acquired academic confidence to meet assignment requirements and an ability to connect theory to their clinical practice. In addition, these six students had also changed their attitudes to theory and perceived it to be an important part of their roles as professional nurses. Theory was seen to constitute knowledge which, in turn, enabled them to be active participants in the care of patients/clients. Despite lacking confidence, Cathy also experienced a change in attitude and demonstrated an appreciation for the role of knowledge in autonomous practice. Carol, however, continued to lack confidence in her academic abilities even though none of her assignments in the Branch Programme was referred. She also disliked the theoretical aspects of the Course and continued to be unmotivated and uninterested in theory. However, she was able to apply theory to practice in the Branch Programme and work independently using her knowledge to support and justify the care she gave.

Cathy's and Carol's profiles may be seen to be less 'integrated' than their peers, although both satisfactorily completed the Course.

209

Branch Programmes

	Academic Confidence mid-branch	Application of Theory to Practice	Change in Attitude towards Theory	Becoming Independent through Knowledge
Ben	Yes	Yes	Yes	Yes
Clare	Yes	Yes	Yes	Yes
David	Yes	Yes	Yes	Yes
Marie	Yes	Yes	Yes	Yes
Paula	Yes	Yes	Yes	Yes
Sarah	Yes	Yes	Yes	Yes
Cathy	No	Yes	Yes	Yes
Carol	No	Yes	No	Yes

Perceptions of nursing in the CFP

Watson and Lea (1997) demonstrated differences in perceptions of caring between male and female student nurses and Watson, Deary and Lea (1999) found differences in perceptions between older and younger student nurses. Using a Caring Dimensions Inventory (Lea, Watson and Deary, 1998) data were gathered at entry to nurse education and after twelve months. However, the researchers acknowledge that the results could be susceptible to 'cohort effects' (p1229) which could be overcome using a longitudinal study.

Several authors share the view that personal identity depends upon the socially enforced theory of Self, by which a human being situates him/herself and acts according to others (Harre, 1983; McCall and Simmons, 1978; Schlenker, 1980; Stringer and Bannister, 1979). For Kelly (1991) personal identity is fashioned by discerning consistent patterns of similarities and differences between oneself and others. These similarities and differences represent 'role constructs' by which we relate ourselves to and distinguish ourselves from others in our social environment. In order to socialise individuals into the role of the nurse, uniform brings with it an aura of cleanliness, sobriety and trustworthiness, which coincidentally, the authors say, acts as a social control over patients. They believe that it signifies both the quasi-religious image and para-military authority of nursing. However, they predicted that the personal freedom of most student nurses would increase as they became part of a university system of general education.

The frustrations of not wearing uniform in the first six months of the Course was apparent in conversations with the younger students in this study. Marie, Sarah, Clare, Paula and Carol all commented on the need to wear uniform to 'feel' like a nurse and gain a sense of identity. In contrast, the mature students felt uncomfortable in uniform. Ben claimed to feel like an imposter; David considered he did not have the knowledge to warrant wearing it and Cathy experienced uniform as having a negative effect, often tempting her to revert to the auxiliary role.

Donaldson (1992) identifies three different types of construct mode, within Kelly's personal construct theory. The intellectual construct mode where intellect and cognition dominate which would, for instance, account for construct modification as a result of gaining theoretical knowledge; the value-sensing construct mode, which I would interpret as being characterised by feelings and values, how to conduct oneself responsibly in clinical practice and learned patterns of acceptable social

211

behaviour, probably more associated with an affective domain, and the core construct mode as Donaldson calls it, refers to those central constructs in which thought and feeling are intermingled. Relating feelings and beliefs about uniform and how each student perceives it could be interpreted using this framework. Particularly relevant in this instance, I believe, is the value-sensing construct mode. It appears that the younger students needed to situate themselves within the institution in order to be of value. This is considered to be a developmental stage (Kegan, 1996) whereby individuals seek a collective so that they belong and consequently shun individuality. Donaldson's analysis implies that we engage in different modes of consciousness and that there are varying ranges and quality of conscious experience for different individuals. The mature students could be said to be formulating their feelings about the wearing of uniform from within an intellectual construct mode, because from this position one would assume that an individual in uniform has earned the right to wear it through acquisition of knowledge.

During an early conversation, Ben implied that he was not 'doing' nursing and that he was looking forward to the Branch Programme which *will give us an opportunity to catch up on nursing experience that we lost during the first eighteen months*. This perception appears to stem from the belief that community, mental health and learning disability placements were not 'nursing'.

It is thought that during the early stages of joining any occupation, the individual sees what the organisation is like and attempts to become a participating member of it (Feldman, 1976; Porter, Lawler and Hackman, 1975; van Maanen, 1976). But, it is extremely difficult for students in the CFP to participate in care within a community, mental health or learning disabilities environment if they do not perceive that it is nursing. During the CFP, it appeared that students were separated from where they perceived the daily tasks of their future role took place [ie. on hospital wards], which led to ambivalence about what was being learned. It is possible that this was a reason for students becoming demotivated to learn. Mortimer and Simmons (1978) believe that with an 'apprenticeship' system it is more likely that the relevance of what is taught is clear, because the learning occurs where the occupational task is performed.

In his one-to-one interview David claimed that he could not *wait to get started* implying that he too perceived the Branch Programme to be the time when nursing would be learned. He believed that hands-on nursing meant that an individual could make a difference, but that as students they could not. Expectancy theory (Mortimer and Simmons, 1978) attaches great importance to the individual's expectations regarding the behavioural outcomes of their efforts and the response to those efforts. On an idealistic level, the reward is that individuals make a contribution to society and make a difference to the lives of certain people.

Changing Branch Programmes

About 18 months ago, I thought that I needed to nurse as all the books say, that is, I needed to develop techniques of nursing. I have since realised that it is only by being my true self, through self awareness, that I can help others. There is a fine line between personal and professional development in nursing.

(David, end of Course questionnaire)

There was ample evidence to suggest a change in students' constructions of nursing practice. Three of my eight participants transferred from general adult nursing to the mental health branch of the Course during the last few months of the CFP as a result of a gradual awakening, a realisation that the role of the nurse did not only extend to physical care within an institutional setting. They began to appreciate that nursing permeates all aspects of life - in the community, in the workplace and in leisure facilities, which means that student nurses have a whole range of options. Unfortunately, sometimes this realisation happens too late in the Course to be able to satisfy the students' changing career aspirations. Students at the time this study was conducted were pressured to choose their Branch Programme at selection interview, prior to understanding the diverse nature of the nurse role. At the centre in which this study was conducted there was limited opportunity for students to transfer Branch Programmes as all places were funded by the Trusts who determined how many qualified nurses they would require from each Branch Programme at the end of the three year period. Ben, David and Sarah were fortunate in that some students from the mental health branch programme had left the Course during the CFP, leaving room for them to transfer. Ben originally chose the general adult branch of nursing prior to commencing the Course because he believed it would be exciting; similar to his work with the mountain rescue and first aid which he enjoyed so much, and consistent with his mother's and friend's experiences as general nurses. Early mental health and learning disabilities placements *horrified* Ben because he had not considered them to be part of nursing. I recognised his intrigue with mental health during the RepGrid interview where he had

213

reported feeling a *growing tolerance* for people with mental health problems. His 'loner' type of personality appeared to suit the one-to-one therapeutic relationship which was often demanded in a mental health care environment and he found the challenge of caring for mentally vulnerable people rewarding. It is interesting to compare his 'previous life' in the military to his chosen speciality branch of mental health nursing; the authoritarian, ordered life of a soldier in contrast to the unpredictable working day in a mental health environment; wearing uniform in the military and often not being able to differentiate by dress between staff and clients in a mental health setting; having order, routines, rules and regulations in military life compared to an often disordered, client-determined, 'out of control' environment in mental health nursing. Ben conveyed his own surprise at the change in himself and how he had adapted to the different way of life in nursing. He often portrayed the lonely life of the soldier and military policeman where no intimacies could be chanced. This, he reported, bred a self-dependence and prevented him from forming friendships. Being a student nurse had called for a completely different approach, where trust and respect for others, who were not in a position of power but in one of vulnerability, were encouraged. Ben commented that his change to mental health from general adult nursing had developed as a growing realisation throughout the CFP; he believed that he had been *indoctrinated* by his family to pursue the *medical* side of nursing. Experiences in the CFP such as people repeatedly being admitted to the Accident and Emergency Department having taken an overdose; counselling dying people whilst out with the Macmillan nurses and wanting to be a part of therapy for people with mental health illness, motivated Ben to change Branch Programme.

Unlike Ben, David did not give any indication at our meetings during early stages of the CFP that he might be more interested in mental health nursing than the general adult branch, although he did refer to general nursing as 'boring' and I remember defending my own general nursing roots. However, his Present Tense Commentaries and episodes submitted in the Reflective Practice Portfolio are all about mental health issues and experiences with mental health clients. Although not obvious in the material I collected, it might be that David developed his interest gradually. There is evidence to suggest that he enjoyed initiating one-to-one relationships with clients, where he could *make a difference* to their lives. He also mentioned early in the CFP that the brain and its aetiology held a fascination for him. Although he does not explicitly say so, I believe he found dealing with people who had 'unusual' patterns of behaviour challenging and this is evident in his choice of scenarios for the Present Tense Commentaries and Reflective Practice Portfolio. Like Ben, David had been exposed only to general nursing prior to the Course and therefore had a rather narrow perspective at that time.

Sarah began to discuss the variety and challenge within nursing during the RepGrid encounter and this, of course, enabled her shift from general adult nursing to the mental health branch. The traditional image of the nurse being based on a ward eroded, but she recognised that this construct had evolved during her nursing auxiliary work on a general medical and neuro-surgical ward when she believed she was giving 'basic care'. During the Branch Programme she told me that there was no such thing as basic care because caring for someone was made up of many elements and each individual had to be viewed in totality. Her construct of nursing had, in Kelly's terms, dilated following her recognition of the complexity of the job. Rather than 'doing to' patients, Sarah demonstrated in her discussions an empathic approach to patient care in which she developed the attitude 'what would it be like if it were me?'. Early in the CFP she talked about *giving a bit of myself* in a counselling session. It appears from the interview conducted six months into the Course that she had a significant experience where she was involved in counselling women with mental health disorders which had considerable influence upon her decision to change Branch Programmes. She commented; *I was buzzin' all day because I had reached these women.*

Similarly to these three students who changed from adult general to mental health nursing, students in Manninen's (1998) study increasingly viewed nursing as a psycho-social and professional activity rather than a technical activity.

Student nurse perceptions of ordinary students

Ben, Carol, Clare and Paula explicitly stressed the difference between being a student nurse and being an 'ordinary' student in a university. At the time that this study was conducted the participants were in their third year of nurse education when the then College of Nursing amalgamated with a university. They had few shared facilities with other higher education students and it was apparent that none of the nursing students mixed with those from higher education, despite the opportunity and having previously complained that everything was *nursey, nursey, nursey.* Being a student nurse meant that individuals were isolated from the facilities available to 'ordinary' students, whether by choice or by restrictions of the institution. Isolation occurred for several reasons; distance between the nursing college and the main university site; student nurses were attending placements which occupied much of their time; their perception that they had additional responsibilities compared to 'ordinary' students; and not having standard university vacations. Paula was adamant that the contrasts between the roles and responsibilities of 'ordinary' students and student nurses should be made explicit. *If you tell people you're a student, they just think she's a student ... I'd rather say I'm a student nurse.* It appears to be insulting to be called a student because of the perceived reputation of mainstream students. Paula emphasised that the Project 2000 course was not an ordinary college course. Carol and Sarah found that friends at university believed student nurses did not have as much academic work to complete, and expected them to have a summer vacation and time off during each working week, as ordinary students do. Clare said that being an ordinary student meant that you would be *spoon fed* and *hand in essays one day and get it back the next* (one-to-one interview). She drew comparisons between herself as a student nurse and her brother who was at university studying for an engineering degree. She told of her frustrations at not having similar recognition as her brother, from her parents.

In addition, the college at that time, tried to impress upon student nurses that they should be able to enjoy the benefits of being a student, and yet on the other hand, the student nurses received messages from their placements that they must arrive on an early shift by 7.30am, even if they had transport or child care problems. But Carol insisted that she would not want to be associated with 'ordinary' students, neither would she want any of the existing modules for student nurses integrated into mainstream higher education, to share with other students.

This construct of 'nurse education' can be seen to differ considerably between student, practitioner and educationalist and some of these issues have already been addressed in Chapter 4.

Belonging and being valued in the Branch Programmes

Unlike Melia (1987), who implied that her student nurses were more concerned with adapting to current situations than preparing to take on the qualified role at some future date, there is evidence in my material which demonstrates the frustrations of students when qualified staff did not give tuition and supervision concerning the everyday responsibilities of being in charge;

I really want to be with this staff nurse; I want to think about the role of staff nurse and find out how to prioritise my day. But she has disappeared ... I feel stressed. Basically I just carry on giving basic care.

(Cathy, Present Tense Commentary)

The task was delegated to me inappropriately. I was not briefed or supported after the incident. Both nurses were my superiors which made it difficult for me to assert myself at a time when I should have had supervision.

(Clare, Ref. Prac. Port.)

For Heidegger (p422) 'everydayness' implies a familiarity in which the individual strives for a natural horizon; a known baseline from which all activity develops. Quite simply, this is exactly what the students were aiming to achieve - a preparedness for the future as a staff nurse. These 'core role structures' as Kelly (p909) calls them are related to expectations of other people to provide a frame of reference for our own construction of our roles so that we can sustain a position within the context in which we intend to function. By construing others, we apparently elaborate upon our constructions of ourselves and this clarifies personal identity and interpersonal relationships (Bannister, Fransella and Agnew, 1971 p99). For my student participants a significant aspect of 'being a nurse' and becoming independent was the acceptance by their colleagues, whether nurses or others in the multidisciplinary team, that they had a place within the practical scheme of activities.

Maslow (1970) identifies 'belonging' within his framework of human needs and acknowledges that individuals strive to satisfy the need to find identification within groups. The importance of being accepted by nursing and multidisciplinary teams was demonstrated mainly through the Present Tense Commentary material, although students also chose scenarios associated with belonging in their Reflective Practice Portfolios. Much of the material relating to this theme emerged from experiences during the CFP where students reported situations where they felt they did not 'belong' and felt 'undervalued'.

To illustrate an extreme of not feeling valued, David recalled his experiences on his first placement where he felt that everyone, without exception, 'treated him like dirt'. He believed that auxiliaries to staff nurses treated him with contempt and this brought with it a degree of misery and discomfort. At about the same time in 1994 I was also informed that one of our students, but not in my study cohort, had had a staff nurse spit on her because she was undertaking a Project 2000 course. This scenario illustrates the worst possible environment in which a student could be expected to function.

Marie reported an incident during the CFP where she was ignored by doctors during a consultant ward round. It was during her first medical ward placement and she says that she was 'allowed' to take charge of the consultant ward round. She described how the doctors were talking amongst themselves, perusing the notes, but ignoring her, even though she had appropriate information about the patients allocated to her. One of the doctors continued to look around for a qualified member of staff despite Marie's insistence that she could provide the information. This episode resulted in Marie feeling inadequate, angry, isolated and inferior. Her reflections included an analysis of her actions and a conclusion relating to her own lack of assertiveness and poor communication skills. Being under-valued in this instance, clearly related to how doctors perceived the student nurse role and the student's ability to adopt a role usually occupied by a qualified member of staff. For me, the issue is also related to common courtesy and how one group of individuals perceive the work and status of another. This dissonance between the perceived roles of carers and curers is traditional and is also derived from socialisation strategies within medical school (Becker, Geer, Hughes and Strauss, 1961).

Subtle actions in clinical practice transfer the message that student nurses should know their place. Carol talked me through an episode in her Present Tense Commentary which related to being undervalued by the nursing team - a simple and frequently practised behaviour;

The night nurse is handing over and there's not enough seats. I'm standing up - all the trained nurses are sitting down and the students are standing up. I feel obliged to stand up.

(Carol, Present Tense Commentary)

More positive experiences were conveyed during the Branch Programme concerning the way students were being accepted into clinical practice by their qualified colleagues. In contrast to this experience in the CFP, Carol talked about her experience during specialist rostered service in operating theatres during the Branch Programme;

When I was working in theatres, you were viewed as someone quite valuable, you know - 'Carol can scrub up and she can assist you'. It was nice to have a bit of trust.

(Carol, Present Tense Commentary)

218

Cathy felt valued because she was introduced as an equal colleague by her health visitor during a teaching session for mothers in a playgroup. She commented, *everyone looks approvingly and is smiling and is encouraging. It's about being valued.* Sarah remembered an occasion where she returned to a placement and the staff nurse said "we're glad you're back, isn't it brilliant to have you back" and "we think you're great and the clients have been asking after you". Clare remembered how important it was for her at all stages to feel useful because to be able to do something meant that you were valued as part of the team. This could be associated with students feeling less valued in the CFP than in the Branch Programme where they had additional knowledge and skills to contribute.

These stories consolidate my interpretations thus far about the segregation between the CFP and the Branch Programme and the meanings that students assign to those periods of their nurse education.

Paterson, Crawford, Saydak, Venkatesh, Tschhikota and Aronowitz (1995), Shead (1991) and White (1996), refer to roles and role conflict experienced by student nurses as part of the socialisation process. In summary, these studies identify conflicts for students relating to feeling pressured by work, job satisfaction, ability, and conflict resolution. They do not however address the issues identified by students in my study, that is, the contrasting identities of being a student/being a nurse.

Temporality as a Heideggerian concept

Through having a perception of what time is and how entities which manifest themselves to us during our existence transpire we develop what Heidegger calls "within-time-ness" (Heidegger, p278). He also calls time an horizon which implies that it is a milestone, a landmark or a scale by which we mark events and give some structure to our lives, although in everyday usage of the word horizon might also imply something which is always ahead or behind, but never reached.

Heidegger explains his interpretation of the fundamental analysis of Dasein and how 'being' is set within Temporality as having a "potentiality for", an authenticity of experience and ultimately, a "being-towards-death" (p276). Whilst Heidegger's chapters concerning temporality in association with death, 'the meaning of care', and the authenticity of 'potentiality-for-being', are interesting and pertinent to this study, I have found his later chapters in Division Two of *Being and Time*, namely - "temporality and everydayness" and "temporality and historicality" more useful. Heidegger (p229) also emphasises the familiarity that time has within our understanding and remarks that vocabulary and everyday discourse is affected by temporality because it is characterised in language through the tenses. But he illuminates the elusiveness of the understanding of time, building on the work of Aristotle and Augustine - "Things past and future belong to time. The former are no longer and the latter are not yet". Sartre (1996, p107) however, suggests that time is simply an infinite number of 'nows' and states that the only possible way of studying temporality is to approach it as a totality which has more meaning than viewing it as a distinct entity. My intention in this chapter has been to situate the students' experiences in context during their development, so that their changing constructs of what the Course and nursing meant to them can be seen in totality. It is not only this chapter which features temporality; the concept is integral to this study in a number of ways, for example, through being conducted over an extended period of time so that both the students' and my own constructs changed. Reflection has enabled experiences to be examined in retrospect, while interpretation, which required a sense of the past, present and future, has allowed participants to contextualise their experiences.

Making sense of changing constructs

Sartre (1996) ontologically relates the past to the present as a result of the "my-ness" of both entities. An individual's past cannot be isolated from the present and is associated with the plurality of Selves, not only in role but in "dimension" (1996, pp106-116). He states that yesterday should be viewed as a transcendence behind our present of today; the past should not be disassociated from us, but rather viewed as part of our development, progress and changing nature. We need to learn to co-exist with what we were. The past appears to give some meaning for present and future events as demonstrated through the fundamental postulate in Kelly's theory of personality.

I concur with Kelly who argues that no one needs to be a victim of their own biography, believing that if an individual wants to change, despite their past, they have the choice to do so. Thus, they have the ability to 'fix' the present. An individual may achieve this through their constructions as being either 'dilation' or 'constriction'. This dimension refers to persons either broadening their view of the world or constricting their view in order to minimise apparent incompatibilities. Dilation can either result in extending personality or in chaos. Constriction may enable the person to become more in control or move

220

towards "an increasingly impoverished world". I would say that generally, students' constructs of nursing during the CFP were constricted in their efforts to defend their perceptions of nursing at the outset of the Course [see Chapter 6]. Because of the incompatibilities experienced during this period constricted constructs were employed in an effort to minimise them and eventually, on reaching the Branch Programmes, students' horizons had broadened as a result of experiences and dilation of their frame of reference. I would argue that the ethos of the Course, at the time of this study, changed during the semester prior to the Branch Programmes commencing, because it suddenly permitted students more freedom to pursue a personal/professional issue for project work and began to prepare students for their chosen nursing speciality. I believe that the Diploma of Higher Education in Nursing Studies course ethos took on a more interpretive approach (Grbich, 1990) to education during the Branch Programmes, encouraging student nurses actively to seek and select experiences which were conducive to the attainment of Course objectives as well as their own agendas. There was less theoretical assessment during the Branch Programme and all assignments were practice-driven rather than subject-driven as had been the case in the CFP. Students spent more time on placements which helped them develop a professional self-image and constantly create new meanings, understandings and definitions of practice situations. This approach to socialisation is thought to encourage and expect a variety of identities including deviant responses, maladaptive outcomes and change (van Maanen, 1976).

To some extent students are still controlled by, for example, the order and statute of the United Kingdom Central Council as Nursing's governing body, the NHS as the potential employer of student nurses while there is also an element of ownership by the university. The structures which govern nursing practice demand that students adhere to determined rules and regulations with regard to their behaviour on placements. Within the Branch Programme they are also encouraged to be creative, self-directed and to explore their thoughts, feelings and attitudes in the learning environment by educators and role models whose purpose it is to nurture a free thinking, innovative reflective practitioner.

The contribution of Kelly's corollaries to understanding temporality

Personal Construct Theory contributes to my interpretations of students' development by providing a perspective on the way that constructs are formed, maintained or changed. Buckenham (1998) stresses that three of Kelly's eleven corollaries have specific application to socialisation into nursing. These corollaries refer to the process of developing constructs through interaction with others, and the way constructs thus become both individual whilst enabling the individual to perform in a role with others.

The Experience corollary within the theory for instance, refers to a person's construction system as varying as the individual successively construes the replication of events. The successive revaluation of events invites the person to place new constructions upon them whenever something unexpected happens. Consequently, they are not static or inflexible. If these modifications were not made one's anticipations would become less and less realistic. Kelly refers to this as a validation process whereby the individual starts with an hypothesis based on previous experience and then tests the hypothesis through subsequent experiences. Experience therefore allows a person to reconstrue and produce more hypotheses. This reconstruing is evident in my participants' accounts and seems to be essential to achieving the desired outcome of becoming a nurse.

The Commonality corollary emphasises that it is the way people construe experiences that makes them similar, not the similarity between the events they experience. This emphasis provides a congruency between personal construct theory and hermeneutic phenomenology in relation to respect for the uniqueness of lived experience.

The Sociality corollary takes account of the nature of other peoples' constructions and so it is a psychology of understandings, but not a psychology of similar undertakings (Kelly, pp66-68). Change in self-construct, like other changes in construct systems, is considered to take place through the experience cycle (Kelly, 1970, 1977) of anticipation, investment, encounter, confirmation or disconfirmation and constructive revision.

Stevens (1996, p162) claims that part of the appeal of Kelly's theory is that it provides a way of understanding people from the outside, that is, the way people make sense of the world and also by providing a means of understanding and gaining access to the standpoint of a particular experiencer.

A construct is described by Kelly as being a "reference axis devised for establishing a personal orientation toward the various events encountered" (Kelly, p11), and this has become evident in my continuous striving to understand the students' perspective from my

222

own. The basis of the assumption of personal construct theory is that;

> Whatever nature may be, or howsoever the quest for truth will turn out in the end, the events we face today are subject to as great a variety of constructions as our wits will enable us to contrive.
>
> (Kelly, 1970, pp1-2)

This reminded me that all perceptions are open to question and reconsideration, and that many everyday experiences can be utterly transformed if we construe in different ways.

Summary

Students had different trajectories through the Course, depending on their pre-Course perceptions, how they had been encouraged or discouraged, who they had made contact with, their personality and disposition, what they perceived the nurse role to be and how they coped with everyday experiences during the nurse education programme. In particular they found 'being a student - being a nurse' simultaneously remarkably confusing, frustrating and demanding. This dual citizenship made life complicated and often resulted in fragmentation of the total educational experience. Conveniently, Kelly provides a corollary which helps to explain these discrepancies of experience, and one which I think should be added to Buckenham's (1998) list of corollaries relevant and applicable to nurse socialisation. The Fragmentation corollary, recognises that a person's construction system is continually in a state of flux. It takes into account that any individual may employ a number of subsystems which might appear to be incompatible with each other and this can produce problems with consistency.

This chapter has attempted to identify the important construct of 'being a student - being a nurse' and how, during the Course, the components of this construct changed. Apart from developing an integrated approach to the theory aspect of the Course during the Branch Programme, students increasingly viewed nursing as a psycho-social activity rather than a technical [skills based] activity.

It appears that various socialisation theories can provide a framework through which an analysis of my data could be facilitated. However, there is no single theory that incorporates or captures all the essences contained within the students' experiences.

Using hermeneutic phenomenology has enabled me to gain some insight into the ways in which students' constructs were changing and at roughly what stage of the Course. Personal construct theory has also enhanced my understanding of the ways in which students construed experiences over time.

In Chapter 10, the Heideggerian concept of 'active subject' is used as a framework to discuss the characteristics of confidence, familiarity and assertiveness in decision making and management of care for patients/clients all of which demonstrate the student nurses' development towards becoming active subjects.

10 Becoming an 'Active Subject'

In Chapter 7, Heidegger's concept of 'thrownness' was explored in relation to students' experiences of unpreparedness, bewilderment and unfamiliarity in situations arising from nursing practice. Consequently these experiences resulted in students losing composure and feeling discomfited. Many of these experiences occurred during the early semesters when students were being exposed to the reality of clinical practice and the diversity of the nurse's role. It was evident that varying degrees or extents of thrownness had been experienced, which led me to develop the following taxonomy;-

Level 1 Unsatisfied anticipations - feeling inadequate
Level 2 Feeling fazed - bewilderment
Level 3 Considerable floundering - feelings of hostility
Level 4 Rescuing Self from thrownness
Level 5 Being rescued by others from thrownness

The latter is the most extreme form of thrownness that I could detect in the student data, but there may be other levels to discover. It was evident that students had the response of thrownness to various situations either because of their lack of knowledge or 'equipment ready-to-hand' (Heidegger, p79). Leonard (1989) reminds us that nothing can be encountered without reference to our background understanding and that every encounter entails an interpretation based upon our background. It follows therefore, that if we do not have this 'background' on which to draw, the likelihood of being thrown is increased.

Thrownness complements the understanding of people as 'active subjects', where experiencing is at the core of all human actions. As active subjects, people seek meaning in life and strive to attain goals. Living with purpose, people are the responsible and irreplaceable agents in charge of their lives (Becker, 1992). If thrownness is at one end of the experiencing spectrum, 'active subject' must be at the other.

This chapter constitutes a summary of students' data which aims to place an interpretation upon the concept of 'active subject' which Heidegger alludes to throughout *Being and Time*.

Characteristics of an active subject

My understanding of the concept 'active subject' derived from the students' accounts is that an individual is able to determine and shape outcomes of experience because they have confidence, knowledge and a familiarity with the event. These attributes evolve as a result of exposure to events and activities in clinical practice. Students develop insight into a 'possible Self' which may be derived from imagined roles or states of being (Markus and Nurius, 1986) which, in turn, stem from "individual significant hopes" (p954). The significant hope for the student nurse is that they become a qualified nurse - a realisation that 'what others are now, I could become'. The image is provided by immediate social experiences in clinical practice where role models are possibly the comparisons with which an individual's own thoughts, feelings, characteristics and behaviours are contrasted to those of salient others. This can serve as an incentive for future behaviour and an indication of what can be achieved. I have already provided some insight into the important role of the supervisor [Chapter 8], which demonstrates that the role requires people who are already established in their careers and who are able to facilitate students' practice so that they become aware of the consequences of their actions. Laurent (1988) states that if students participate actively in decision-making and have more responsibility, dependence upon the supervisor is minimised and independence and originality are promoted. A poor supervisor/student relationship is thought to provide a recipe for dependence. The security for students to become 'active subjects' is often provided by a supervisor who is aware of the needs of students. Encouraging students to become more involved in decision making with regard to patient care also has the effect of increasing and maintaining motivation and promoting satisfaction.

Students as active subjects in nursing practice

In her Reflective Practice Portfolio Paula described an episode where her supervisor asked her to teach a patient how to use a patient controlled analgesia system (PCAS). To begin with Paula was concerned about not having time to prepare the session, but her supervisor assured her that she was perfectly capable of providing the necessary information to the patient, and that she would also be present if any important instructions were omitted. This demonstration of confidence in the student resulted in Paula making a decision about her teaching

226

strategy, content of the session, learning checks and evaluation of her own teaching. The patient was able to use the PCA system efficiently post-operatively and this served to enhance Paula's confidence in her ability to teach. Accepting the challenge of being an active subject meant that Paula had to make a choice. The Choice corollary of Kelly's (pp45-47) Personal Construct Theory, acknowledges that a person often chooses between alternatives which provide a greater possibility for extension and definition of their own system. To be an active subject a person must make a choice when confronted with the opportunity to do so. This is where inner turmoil can manifest itself.

> Which shall man [sic] choose, security or adventure? Shall he choose that which leads to immediate certainty or shall he choose that which may eventually give him wider understanding?
>
> (Kelly, p45)

If an individual is willing to tolerate some day-to-day uncertainties then the field of vision, predictions and anticipations may become extended. Paula had to weigh up the possible outcomes of the teaching session, but she was not 'thrown'. She had, apparently, been gradually more and more involved in caring for patients in control of their own analgesia. The supervisor had offered support and encouragement and demonstrated confidence in Paula's ability to undertake the task. In her reflections upon the event Paula stated that student-led seminars had been useful, but she recognised that her peers had often been too kind with their evaluations of her teaching ability. She had some inner turmoil as, in college, she had been taught always to plan before undertaking a teaching session. Responding spontaneously to the demands of clinical practice often requires nurses to be flexible and adaptable. Becoming actively involved in decision-making and spontaneous practice often calls for some degree of compromise. Paula had been present at several similar sessions where her supervisor had imparted information about PCAS to patients. These had occurred spontaneously and the supervisor had demonstrated a confident and competent performance. Within Kelly's Experience corollary (pp50-54), the successive revaluation of events invites a person to place new constructions upon experiences whenever something unexpected happens. This acts as a validation process whereby existing constructions are put to the test of experience. It appears that the 'active subject' emerges when the individual attempts to discover recurrent themes or orderliness in a sequence of events. If this is not achieved, then it could be that experience does not amount to much, other than being just another experience.

Sarah used her previous experience on a placement to anticipate the sequence of events and routine on an acute mental health ward. Kelly refers to this anticipation as a capacity to predict and therefore make experiences more and more manageable (p52). Sarah illuminated the concept of 'active subject' during her Present Tense Commentary;

I am quite worried because it's my first day back to a placement that I've been on before. I look around and everyone's getting on and within seconds, I've decided, right sod this, I'm getting on with things as normal and the meeting starts and someone immediately mentions warm up and I say, "yeh, I'll do that".

(Sarah, Present Tense Commentary)

Taking an active part within the team enabled Sarah to re-enter the ward membership. In turn, this led to acceptance, a feeling of belonging and having value among other nurses. After contributing to the meeting through the 'warm up', Sarah was then welcomed back with positive comments which nourished her confidence, encouraged her to actively participate in the everydayness of the ward and demonstrated a positive regard for her - something she would have been taught to have for others. She already had experience in this environment and enjoyed not having to be told to do things; rather, she used her initiative and relished the responsibility that the qualified staff delegated to her.

The potential personal hazards and difficulties of making predictions based on previous experience have been demonstrated by Ben [see Chapter 7], where he experienced a degree of thrownness after being re-allocated to a ward. He expected the experience to be the same, but during his absence, changes had occurred within the ward team which resulted in his personal turmoil. Sartre (1996, p433) states that to be active involves a conscious intention which finally produces an anticipated result. However, this does not mean that an individual must foresee all the consequences of the act. It appears that there is an element of gamble in being an active subject, as all eventualities cannot possibly be anticipated. Taking a risk or gamble is associated with 'situated freedom' (Becker, 1992), whereby individuals find a balance between complete freedom to do as they please and a complete determinism where activities are governed. Situated freedom means that in any given situation people can make choices. Sartre says that people are condemned to freedom and that even not choosing is an influential choice. It is apparent that individuals confront thrownness and freedom as interpersonal relationships are negotiated and co-constitution of meaning is developed. Becker (1992) refers to this as an 'existential a priori' - a fact of life.

Thrownness also constitutes other facts of life such as loneliness, anxiety, meaninglessness and unfinished actualisation. The opposite of these, which I associate with being an active subject, are relatedness, security, meaningfulness and self-actualisation. In clinical nursing practice, self-actualisation appears to occur when other corresponding existentials are satisfied; that is, that students have support, security in the environment and encouragement, which raise their self-esteem. Potentially, becoming an active subject could emerge at any time during the Course, but participants in this study demonstrated cognitive and behavioural activities associated with becoming 'active' mainly in the Branch Programme, although potentially, thrownness and active subject may co-exist. There is evidence from early stages of the study to suggest that students were being active subjects, but in an auxiliary role. That is, they were making decisions about activities which did not require a knowledge base. This has, to some extent, been discussed in Chapter 6 where I introduced the hermeneutic concept of 'intentionality'. It may be, then, that individuals can be 'active subjects' at different levels of functioning.

In order to make the role transition from student to staff nurse more successful, Alavi, Cooke and Crowe (1997) designed the third year curriculum of a Bachelor of Nursing programme to include elements of nursing practice commensurate with the expected ability of a staff nurse. Their research demonstrated that where holistic care, time management, prioritisation of care, working as a team member and sophisticated clinical reasoning were introduced as deliberate strategies in students' learning the transition to the workplace was more effective. These appear to be key areas in which staff nurses need to be active subjects. However, there are constraints on just how much an individual can be an active subject. The UKCC Code of Professional Conduct (1992) contains explicit clauses which relate to professional accountability and responsibility. Particularly relevant to being an 'active subject' are clauses two and four;

> ensure that no act or omission on your part, or within your sphere of responsibility, is detrimental to the interests, condition or safety of patients and clients.
>
> (UKCC, 1992, clause two)

and

acknowledge any limitations in your knowledge and competence and decline any duties or responsibilities unless able to perform them in a safe and skilled manner.

(UKCC, 1992, clause four)

Commitment to being an active subject

Working within this broad remit provides some scope for professional practice and deepens commitment through action. Part of the existential Self is formed through commitment; Carol demonstrated her commitment to the project of managing a ward in her Reflective Practice Portfolio. Part of being an active subject involved the prioritisation of care, and recognition of which patients required urgent or special attention. Often the patients whom she perceived as requiring this urgent attention needed contributions from other disciplines. For example, Carol made it her business to ensure that patients who were going to operating theatre, needed specialist care, required investigations in X-ray or who had to be seen by the consultant were attended to before those who could manage independently. Even arranging meal breaks called for insight into skill mix as did the ability to handle unexpected occurrences. Carol described what Heidegger (p33) refers to as the core existentials in her reflective account and commented on the sense of security she gained from the ward sister, the respect she felt the qualified staff afforded her whilst in the ward manager role, and her raised self-esteem when individuals evaluated her performance very positively. To conclude her reflections, Carol acknowledged how she had been informed by the experience and the limitations of her abilities during this management exercise and how her weaknesses could be addressed. Through these insights she subsequently managed several wards as a student and stated that each episode became more and more 'comfortable'. This response to an ever-changing identity, from a Heideggerian perspective, is referred to as 'living authentically'. This means that an individual does not arrive at a static state, but continues in an upward spiral toward constructing the Self (Knowles, 1986). The process is thought to enable people to grow increasingly self-reflective and to live in accord with values and beliefs. Becker (1992, p94) acknowledges that we get to know ourselves through commitment, because it tends to take us beyond our current identities to develop new and desired ways.

In college, situations are created where students can practise the role of active subject so that they gain experience in a safe and controlled

230

environment. Presenting projects, teaching peers and joint presentations are an expected part of being a student nurse. It is commonplace for unexpected interruptions and unanticipated problems to affect the smooth running of these planned sessions which subsequently demand that students problem solve, negotiate and compensate for these eventualities. But, rather than being thrown by such an event [and recalling it as a catastrophe], students in the later stages of the Course met the challenge and used it as a learning opportunity to determine and shape a particular desired outcome.

Active subject or 'expert'?

In Chapter 8, Clare portrayed herself as an active subject whilst caring for a patient with a heroin addiction. Her commitment to advocate for her patient resulted in a change of, and improvement in, care - a desirable outcome of being an active subject.

Benner (1984) might classify Clare's behaviour as 'proficient' within her 'novice to expert' taxonomy of clinical skill competence because the behaviour satisfies the given criteria. The five stages that Benner presents incorporate performance characteristics at each level of development and aim to identify the teaching/learning needs at each level. A proficient nurse [stage 4 of the taxonomy], perceives situations as 'wholes', rather than as 'aspects' and is able to perceive the meaning of the situation in terms of long-term goals and outcomes. Clare wrote convincingly of her understanding of Entonox and the research she had read. Her decision to be an advocate for the patient stemmed from an understanding of what might happen if he did not receive analgesia. Her reflections also included detailed consideration of options available and possible outcomes of these actions.

It is my interpretation that a nurse can be at any of Benner's stages at any one time, depending on the situation. One could be a novice in a counselling situation, but an expert in caring for an individual receiving life support. My criticism of Benner's taxonomy relates to the way in which it has been used uncritically by nurses, to represent learning and performance across the board as a staged process, especially in applying it to the development of the student nurse undertaking an initial education programme. I believe that a student can only ever become an 'expert' student, because they have not had the experience necessary to understand the intricacies of expert practice, which Benner describes as "having a deep understanding of the total [nursing] situation" (p32).

Perhaps then, Clare performed at a 'proficient student' level, rather

231

than as a 'proficient practitioner'. In addition, she was unable to action her suggestion to use Entonox because, by virtue of the rank of student nurse, she was unable to actually do anything about the patient's pain. However, she did make a decision to advocate for the patient and this required anticipation of a desired goal.

Being an active subject requires creativity

Ben decided, at the last minute, to scrap a lesson plan he had devised prior to teaching his peer group about client-centred therapy. He reported feeling confident about his presentation, having read extensively around the subject and feeling more comfortable with an alternative approach to teaching than he had originally planned. This spontaneity resulted from a hunch that his chosen methods were unsuitable for the student group. Ben thought he had been aiming to satisfy an agenda dictated by the college, rather than adopting a strategy relevant and appropriate for his student group. Being able to recognise this and actively install another strategy, demanded confidence and conviction. Ben claimed that his personal goal was to involve the other students in an experiential style learning activity rather than a didactic situation which, he stated, *would fail to reach the group with the same intensity*. Ben acknowledged that he did not give himself time to reflect before further action, which Ashcroft and Foreman-Peck (1994, p72) say is essential for the novice. Rather, he chose a more flexible, imaginative and improvisatory approach. Creativity is thought to be an intentional act that is open to the not yet known or formed (Miller, 1981). It involves being willing to take a step in a process, wherever it leads, and then actively taking another step. Being an active subject in this kind of situation involves taking a risk, but feeling secure and confident enough to predict the likely outcome.

The stories that students told and which I have identified as defining an 'active subject' have arisen from the desire to make sense of their environment and choose suitable actions which enhance the care given to patients and clients. In 1980, Louis used the term 'sense making' to describe the process of integration into an occupation and its institutional norms. According to Louis individuals can cope with everyday events without undue surprise for much of the work undertaken in as little as six months after entering a nursing course. Bradby (1990) confirmed these findings and stated that students felt more comfortable with clinical areas and had grasped theoretical concepts by this time. The participants in my study did not demonstrate

232

'comfort' in all the clinical areas where they were placed, nor did they demonstrate an understanding of the basic theoretical concepts until they had entered the Branch Programme. Some developed an awareness and understanding before others - indeed, there is no evidence to suggest that they all developed at the same rate. Each participant, depending on their experience, maturity, interest and the placement, learned and developed at a different rate and at different times during the Course. However, there is the need for students to make sense of their situations before they can become active subjects.

Gray and Smith (1999) report on a study of the professional socialisation of student nurses undertaking the Diploma of Higher Education in Nursing Studies course in Scotland. They identified five phases through which student nurses pass before they become staff nurses. Being an active subject, that is, demonstrating problem-solving skills and decision making, are referred to indirectly when the authors describe management skills, assertiveness and confidence. However, there is no acknowledgement that individuals developed at different rates and the ultimate phase - "the end is nigh" (p644) represents the experience of all participants. As the students in my study demonstrated their ability to be 'active subjects' at various stages of the Course, albeit mostly in the Branch Programme, I would argue that familiarity with the environment, experience and the student/supervisor relationship [support systems] are some of the major influences upon the ability of students to be 'active'. It does not 'just happen' in the last semester.

Day, Field, Campbell and Reutter (1995) reported the findings of their socialisation study of nurses according to whether students were in their first, second, third or fourth year. They found that third year students were no longer totally bound by rules; they had begun to discern how and when to apply them in a particular context. In their fourth year students recognised the importance of becoming politically active in order to change the system and demonstrated a concern for processes and outcomes.

Maslow's *Hierarchy of Needs* (Crain, 1992; Maslow, 1968; Maslow, 1970) identifies self-actualisation as the ultimate need which individuals strive to satisfy. It is a concept associated with motivation and the fulfilment of one's potentials, capacities and talents. In order to achieve self-actualisation, the other four needs must be met. Maslow's theory is essentially phenomenological in that it reveres the Self, rather than the environment or society as the motivating force. It appears from the students' stories, illuminating the concept of 'active subject', that self-actualisation and the desire for personal and professional growth are inextricably linked. Setting goals, feeling secure in the environment,

233

nourishing self-esteem and belonging to a team, are needs to be satisfied before students are able to take on the responsibility of making decisions and advocating fully for patients and clients. Once the basic requirements have been met, students aim to fulfil their potential within the team. It becomes less important to conform to all the rules, regulations and guidelines and more important to use creativity, intuition and sophisticated reasoning (Alavi et al. 1997; Benner, 1984).

Summary

The confidence to be able to self-actualise and become an active subject may emerge at any time, particularly during the Branch Programmes, regardless of whether students are undertaking the adult general or mental health branches. This chapter has demonstrated how being an 'active subject' equates with personal and professional development, but not necessarily with arriving at the end of the Course.

'Active subject' was portrayed in the students' stories where decision making, advocating for patients and clients and a desire to be heard were of paramount importance to the student. 'Active subject' and 'thrownness' could be considered as bi-polar constructs whereby one is a desirable characteristic of the qualified nurse and the other is not. Parallels have been drawn between the Choice and Experience corollaries in Kelly's Personal Construct Theory and the Heideggerian concept of 'active subject'.

To bring Part IV to an end, my student participants' perceptions of themselves and their professional development has been captured in verse, which I have scripted from the students' letters as they left the Course to take up their staff nurse positions around the country. Unfortunately, Clare did not complete the final data collection phase and so there is no poem to complete her story. Despite efforts I was unable to trace her. However, this is the only data set missing from a total of fifty-six sets [eight students each with seven data sets], and I consider myself fortunate to have achieved this.

234

Mystories (2)

Ben

You told me I could do it,
and guess what - you were right!
When I think of how I was then -
self-centred, egotistical, militaristic,
I can hardly believe it myself.
I wouldn't change a single moment though,
because it's all made me a better nurse.
The first day I was wearing a suit and tie and wondering
what the hell the others were doing in jeans and tee shirts.
There have been times when I wanted to pack it all in;
times when I felt angry and powerless.
Every time I finished an assignment or placement,
I was given a lift to 'climb the next hill'.
New friends I've shared good times with,
plenty of laughter and tears.
I have learned that I can rely on others but
retain my individuality.
You would not recognise me -
I dress differently, look different and talk differently.
Where I used to be authoritarian and militaristic,
I am now strictly democratic and chilled out.
My total outlook on life has changed.
I know, and can work with, my imperfections.
The big wide world awaits and I'm terrified.
Working in such a stressful environment will mean that support systems
will be well established.
I've a feeling I'll need it.
Next time I see you, it's your round.

Carol

Well it's pretty difficult to sort out three years of experiences and feelings.
I don't remember ever having a blinding flash of inspiration,
it was more of a gradual process.
My first day on the Course, I was very self-conscious and naive.
My first placement was nerve wracking -
"why the hell am I here" and "what the hell am I doing?".
I started to get disillusioned and the assignments were a nightmare.
I had to learn how to study and write essays again,
it took a lot of willpower.
It all sounds like doom and gloom, but I had positive feedback
from placements, where I never had a problem.
I made some really good friends - it was sad to leave the nurses' home.
Friends and family have really helped me through the Course.
After a busy day at work,
the prospect of a night studying was thoroughly depressing.
There were times when I could have jacked it all in
and done something mindnumbing and easy!
This has been the biggest challenge of my life.
Now it's a great sense of relief
but also a great sense of loss.
It's difficult to relax - I should be doing something.
I'm very happy, but there is still so much to learn,
the responsibility can be overwhelming.
Enough about me, write soon ...

Cathy

There is more to nursing than you think!
Looking back I couldn't have managed without my friends
as there was no practical help available for children at college.
I felt motivated, excited, happy - I had status - a student nurse.
I was conscientious and worked hard and did the best I could.
Forty-one per cent knocked my confidence -
where did I go wrong?
The assignments caused so much grief,
placements and studying was stressful.
Results being posted for all to see was torture!
I really valued having a tutor - we built up a good working relationship

236

and became friends.
The pace of work in the community was slower and more rewarding,
nurses on busy wards were already too pushed for time.
Group discussions with fellow students,
shared experiences, let off steam and support for each other.
On many occasions on placements,
I felt my contribution was not considered or regarded.
Lack of resources is frustrating
and attitudes of some staff is disheartening.
The morning our final results were posted we were jubilant -
I never thought I would make it.
The responsibility of being a staff nurse is daunting,
but I learn something new every day.
I've applied to do midwifery,
Watch this space ...

David

There I was, happily ambling through life
when I had a revelation - I wanted to be a nurse!
I thought about becoming a doctor,
but as I didn't think I was a God, this notion soon passed by.
A placement in a day centre made me change direction,
from adult general nursing to mental health.
It was the best decision I could have made.
There were occasions when I nearly quit the Course -
When I was given one day off for the birth of my daughter,
just after we had had a lecture on 'paternity leave'!
Again when I was told not to mix socially with clients, and
when a vacancy came up at the Haagan Daas cafe in town.

There is this theory that we are all alike -
same dreams, ambitions etc. Bollocks!
I feel that I have done this despite college attitudes,
not because of them.
The main reason for continuing is simply that I enjoy it
and I'm bloody good at it.
I can put my hand on my heart and say that
I have no fears in relation to becoming a staff nurse.
They say that self-awareness is the most important thing
you learn on this Course.

237

I'm confident that I already possessed that.
Maybe the most I have gained is knowledge and clinical experience.
With this in mind, maybe I could have done some of this Course
by correspondence.
Yours 'n all that ...

Marie

Hello stranger how are you?
A lot has happened since I saw you last.
Nursing had always been in the back of my mind,
So I decided to do something about it.
I found community work interesting and
counselling was something I had a talent for.
The work was fulfilling and rewarding and
thoroughly enjoyable.
The essays and assignments have been a pain,
not complicated, just time consuming.
I missed my family and I missed Sam.
The support from friends kept me going and
knowing I would have some sort of future.
I am happy, happier than I have ever been.
No-one is going to treat me like dirt any more,
As now I am a staff nurse.
Wish me luck.

Paula

I ran up a huge overdraft
and had real difficulty with the essays.
I think I made things worse for myself,
by getting in a state.
I am getting more and more nervous about
the responsibilities and expectations of being a staff nurse.
I am completely different to when I saw you last -
I am not the shy, quiet girl any more.
I am confident, because I have had to be.
There are times when I feel upset,
but there are plenty of good times as well.
I thought the Course was good -

238

knowing the reasons behind what you do.
I can't wait to have some dosh
and do plenty of clothes shopping.
I'll write again soon, take care ...

Sarah

It seems strange now, watching TV and having the cleanest house,
gone are the part-time jobs to make ends meet.
I qualified as a mental health nurse, I changed from adult general,
it was a tough decision, but the right one.
I grew as a person throughout the Course,
I became more assertive and confident.
But I got third year blues and became ill -
my colleagues seemed not to care, but my family and friends supported
me.
Physically and mentally I was drained,
I had to work twice as hard to catch up.
But I showed everyone - I qualified!

A lot has changed,
I have a new job and a completely different lifestyle.
People actually listen,
but at the end of the day, the buck stops here.
Life starts from here, as the last three years have been on hold.
With all best wishes and kind regards ...

Part V

Discussion and Emergent Issues

In Part IV, Chapters 6 to 10 set out issues raised by students at various points in their development towards becoming nurses. Specifically, these experiences related to 'intentionality' and students' comportment toward the Course and nursing; experiences of 'thrownness' within which I identified levels of severity of being 'thrown'; 'being-in-the-world-with-others' such as other students in accommodation, the student cohort, patients, clients and relatives and supervisors in clinical practice. The Heideggerian concept of 'temporality' was used as a framework to elaborate changes in students' constructs during the Course and finally, experiences where students could be seen to be developing decision-making skills and participating autonomously in clinical practice were considered through the concept of the 'active subject'.

Part V, which consists of this chapter alone, is concerned with emergent issues from the thesis and discussions relating to the specific contributions of the work to both practice and research in nursing and nurse education.

Even as I write up these findings, ontologically, I am still experiencing an interaction with my participants' texts, the text of each chapter, Heidegger's text and my own textual understandings; the hermeneutic circle is still in play.

11 Considerations, Contributions and Closure

My aims for this research, stated in Chapter 1, were twofold; to illuminate experiences of student nurses undertaking the Diploma of Higher Education in Nursing Studies course in an attempt to understand the meaning they assign to those experiences and, through a hermeneutic analysis of their stories, to portray the learning milieu in which students become nurses. These aims were developed from questions which were generated through my reading of associated literature and from my own experiences of being a nurse and nurse educator.

My contributions to knowledge

The findings of my study are related to selection and recruitment of student nurses onto diploma courses in terms of their entry qualifications and literacy skills; whether potential student nurses had previous nursing experience and how this might affect their professional development. I also make a contribution to knowledge with regard to mature students' perceptions and how they develop during the Diploma of Higher Education in Nursing Studies course. The phenomenon of 'being-a-student'/'being-a-nurse' also exposes the dual citizenship of student nurses undertaking current courses and how these sometimes conflicting identities affect professional development. 'Thrownness' has also been identified in students' stories as a potential source of stress in clinical practice. Through an analysis of their stories, I have been able to develop a taxonomy of thrownness which has potential as an educational tool. Experiences associated with death and dying dominate these stories of thrownness and I suggest a way forward in helping students to deal with such experiences. Findings relating to supervision of students in nursing practice contribute to the existing literature, in particular exposure to situations and environments which encourage students to become active subjects. I make a significant contribution to the methodological literature within nursing research through the philosophical approach, data collection and analysis strategies. I also evaluate the role of reflection within the study and how it has contributed to research processes and my own development. Recommendations and actions proposed from my study are emboldened within the text of this chapter.

Entry qualifications and literacy

The participants in my study entered nursing with a variety of academic qualifications. However, most of them lacked confidence in their academic abilities, even though collectively, only two assignments [out of a potential 56] were considered unsatisfactory on first submission. This success rate is different to other cohorts of students undertaking healthcare courses (Holder, Jones, Robinson and Krass, 1999). These researchers found that, despite a high university-entrance requirement in terms of qualifications, literacy problems persisted indicating that exposure to new subjects and different demands upon writing skills, may place those with restricted literacy skills at an academic disadvantage.

Although no generalisations can be drawn from my small sample, there was no connection between my participants, their entry qualifications, academic performance or gender differences. Recognising that students entering nursing do so at different ages and with different backgrounds means that entry pathways into nursing should be flexible and responsive to different levels of knowledge and experience.

Flexibility includes provision of pre-Course or integrated literacy assistance which ideally, should take place before problems and weaknesses affect academic success. However, in a curriculum which is perceived to be dominated by academic work, students may not prioritise their time to deal with weaknesses. Students undertaking the Diploma course at the time that this study was conducted, were assessed on entry to the Course and offered remedial work outside the curriculum. A better approach may be to integrate literacy skills into the curriculum, but this strategy has been criticised in the past for taking up valuable time perceived to be better spent teaching nursing skills. However, it should be acknowledged that within the remit of lifelong learning, adequate literacy training should be given to launch the student on that lifelong journey of learning. Long-term literacy assistance offered for each student cohort might reduce individual tutor's time coaching academically weak students [see Chapter 4].

Previous nursing experience

Traditionally, it has been thought that having previous nursing experience as an auxiliary nurse or care assistant would be beneficial to the individual in understanding the nurse role and in successful socialisation into nursing. The largest, most recent externally funded Project 2000 study (Macleod Clark et al. 1996) did not address possible influences that previous healthcare experience might have upon perceptions of the philosophy and practice of nursing. From my study it can be seen that students may develop an identity with the occupational group of auxiliaries and as a consequence, develop different preconceptions and perceptions of what nurse education entails. Indeed, Cathy, Sarah and Marie commented on experiences where previous experience hindered development of their student nurse role and it may be necessary to break loose from that existing identity before the student can progress and develop a new perspective.

I suggest that in order to refashion their construct of nursing, students with previous nursing experience may need to go through a period of de-skilling in order to learn basics from a different perspective. This issue should be drawn to the attention of those who select potential students and encourage participation in nursing environments prior to starting the Course. There are benefits of feeling comfortable in a healthcare environment, but there is danger that the auxiliary role becomes more 'natural' to the student to the detriment of learning how to become a professional nurse. The differences in purpose, role, responsibility and outcomes of the roles of auxiliary and student may need to be discussed early in the Course so that students can make a distinction between past and current roles and goals. It is evident from my study, that despite having experience in a healthcare environment, an individual is as likely to misconstrue the role of the nurse as someone who has no previous experience. At the time that my study was conducted students were entering nursing with various experiences of healthcare and it was often difficult to assess how competent they had become at some basic nursing skills and also frustrating to them, when their skills were not acknowledged in clinical practice. The Peach Report (UKCC, 1999; 5.37) suggests that training for auxiliaries based upon common standards may improve consistency in the quality of care provision at this level. It might also assist with determining how students, who were once auxiliaries, might transfer skills across and between roles.

Mature students

Despite mature students constituting a third of entrants into nurse education (Seccombe, Jackson and Patch, 1995), Glackin and Glackin (1998) comment that there appear to be no studies of mature and young students working alongside each other on Project 2000 courses and so I have some contribution to make to this aspect of nurse education.

In my study, relationships within the cohort were often strained as a result of age division, perceived irresponsibility toward the Course and feeling intimidated in the large group. Macleod Clark et al. (1996) provide demographic information about their sample depicting proportions of female and male student nurses, age and qualification on entry to the Project 2000 courses, but do not address any of the issues associated with these three variables. Certainly there is no reference to collective or unique experiences of being-with other students in accommodation or differences in perceptions between age cliques. The mature participants in my study valued their life experience and previous occupations in preparing them to deal with various situations in nursing although this was a source of irritation to some of the younger cohort members. Mature students had anxieties about academic work, but this was no more severe than that experienced by the young students. They also appeared to develop a poor self-concept in relation to academic work and perceived that young students were at an advantage because of their more recent study experiences. Whilst there were no differences in academic performance between female and male students, my study suggests that male student nurses may not be given equal consideration in relation to parenting. I recall David's situation, revealed in his letter at the end of the Course, that he was not allowed any paternity leave for the birth of his third child. Similarly, Cathy commented in her letter [evidenced in the poem at the end of Part IV], that there was no provision for child care whilst she was on the Course so that she had to depend upon friends and relatives to fit in with her shifts. In a study conducted by McEvoy (1995) attrition rates amongst students of all ages were primarily a result of personal and domestic, rather than academic circumstances. This suggests that retention of 'mature' students could be improved if pre-registration programmes were more flexible.

In contrast to Smithers and Griffin's (1986) work with higher education students my study participants perceived their cohort to be split into age determined cliques because of similar age-related interests, inside and outside nursing. Yet, on their placements, students of all ages provided support to each other. Segregation by age therefore, only occurred in the college environment where an element of choice of group membership was available. This notion of student's self-division has not been apparent in any of the studies of nurses' socialisation, particularly as many of these tend to report the activities of students on traditional courses where mature students have always been an unacknowledged group. I would argue therefore, that issues relating to mature students in nurse education should be recorded - not to isolate them further, but to ensure that Courses satisfy their needs.

Perceptions of nursing

In Chapter 6 'Intentionality' provided a useful framework through which students' perceptions of nursing and the Course were interpreted. The concept can provide nurse educationalists with some insight into how perceptions of nursing can be reconstructed through knowledge and experience. Understanding students' constructions of nursing and possible ways in which students develop cognitively during the Course could be useful in developing goals and learning outcomes for clinical placements and structuring the important first semester/term of the pre-registration nursing curriculum. I consider it important to acknowledge that a period of adjustment for students at the beginning of the Course, which allows for the interplay between emotions and cognitions experienced in a new learning environment, might be useful as part of the learning process.

I find it interesting that all my study participants shared a traditional image of nursing in preference to more recent ones even when information was imparted to them through leaflets and videos, for instance, produced by the UKCC. I made sense of their perspective using Kelly's Choice Corollary, in which he explains that individuals choose to believe the perception which will confirm expectations. Their expectations included the belief that on community, learning disabilities and mental health placements, they did not observe 'nursing' and therefore experienced difficulty in taking part and identifying role models for their nursing practice. However, these perceptions underwent gradual reconstruction as evidenced by Ben, David and Sarah, who changed Branch Programmes toward the end of the CFP. No other studies have identified the experiences and changes in perception of nursing which might lead to a change in chosen Branch Programme for students undertaking the Diploma of Higher Education in Nursing Studies course. Indeed, I am not aware of it being mentioned in any of the existing socialisation studies. I have identified the changes in constructs of nursing held by the three students who changed Branch Programme resulting from their exposure to challenging, intriguing, personally moving situations which inspired an interest in alternative ways of caring.

The CFP and Branch Programmes

Within my study there were clear distinctions between being-a-student in the CFP and being-a-nurse in the Branch Programmes. This phenomenon of being-a-student, being-a-nurse accompanied the belief that the CFP was a test of stamina, concerned with the theoretical components of the Course, whilst the Branch Programmes constituted the majority of opportunities to learn the desired nurse role. These contrasting and sometimes conflicting identities of being-a-student/being-a-nurse have not been identified in previous research studies concerned with 'becoming' processes of student nurses (eg Macleod Clark et al. 1996; Paterson et al. 1995; Shead, 1991 and White, 1996).

Most pre-registration nursing students select their Branch Programme on entry to the CFP and this is thought to suit the service providers who purchase education on the basis of anticipated human resource requirements in the Branch areas (UKCC, 1999, p29). Seventy per-cent of students are reported to know which Branch they want to pursue at the start of the Course and do not change their minds. The other thirty percent are either unsure or change their minds during the CFP. It might be beneficial therefore, given this high rate of uncertainty, for students to choose their Branch Programme after exposure to a variety of nursing environments at the end of the CFP.

There is a view that fitness to practice is not necessarily being achieved through the current construction of Courses comprising a CFP and Branch Programme and it has been suggested that Course planners should be aware of the implications of a primary-led NHS on the education of nurses (UKCC, 1999, p39). This implies that the Branch Programmes may not even exist in the future. In view of this recommendation, I wonder what will motivate students to undertake a nursing Course, if, as in my study, students perceived the Branch Programmes to be the time when nursing skills were learned. The other alternative which The Peach Report (UKCC, 1999, 2.22) suggests, is that the Branch structure be retained, but for new specialisms to be based upon community or acute and long term care.

My findings associated with perceptions of practice and theory

248

concur with Macleod Clark et al. (1996). Students perceived nursing as a caring profession, with an emphasis on practical and physical work and nursing the sick. The importance of gaining practical experience diminished as the Course progressed, whilst the view that Project 2000 students have a different approach to care assumed a higher profile. Similarly, my students assigned less and less importance to technical skills and more to psycho-social skills as time passed.

My study differs in its value to nurse educators with regard to changing constructs, because with a much smaller sample, I have offered insight into experiences which pre-empted or stimulated a change in construct. Understanding the components of such experiences is useful in identifying aspects of the nurse education curriculum which possibly need modifying or exploring further.

Self-directed study

Exploring and reflecting upon perceptions of nursing and how these perceptions have been acquired in order to deconstruct and reconstruct more accurate perceptions might provide additional 'structure' through which students could become more self-directed. The structure of the Course was found to be important amongst the students in my study. Unless they were clear about the structure and intentions of the Course, they were unsure of their own comportment in relation to it. They appeared to have difficulty with self-directed learning if the structure of the Course appeared fragmented or haphazard. It was not enough to be told that the Course, to a greater extent, was self-directed. Being self-directed requires pacing, effective searching skills, an ability to use resources effectively, a knowledge of systems within the university and knowing how one learns. The ethos for self-directed learning has to be supportive with appropriate strategies in place; otherwise students may become isolated and neglected and their learning is ineffectual. It might also appear that installing a strategy of self-directed learning is a 'cop out' for teachers. Students need clear information about Course content, subject content, arrangement of themes within the curriculum, information and sometimes instruction about being self-directed.

Experiences of 'thrownness'

One of the major original contributions my study makes to nursing and nurse education is the identification of a taxonomy associated with

249

experiences which threaten Self. It was evident that experiences associated with unfamiliarity, fear and threat, either to the personal or professional Self, resulted in thrownness; a concept described by Heidegger (p79) as a lack of 'equipment ready to hand'. These situations frequently occurred in clinical practice during the CFP and sometimes in the Branch Programme. Although the taxonomy was developed from student nurses' experiences, it could be applied to qualified nurses' experiences and indeed, to other disciplines outside healthcare. As 'thrownness' appears to be a new concept within nursing practice and nurse education, I believe it warrants exploration on a more general and larger scale. I intend to collect experiences of thrownness from students and qualified nurses through diaries of critical incidents and to collate them thematically. Analysis of the incidents may challenge or confirm my taxonomy, but these incidents have the potential to indicate where attention should be drawn in order to prepare and educate nurses to deal with potentially 'threatening' situations. The potential of such a study could be linked with clinical supervision and the development of practice portfolios and reflective practice. As all participants in my study had at least one experience of 'thrownness' to portray, I might assume that students would appreciate some support mechanism to assist with their development through such an experience. The thrownness taxonomy could also be strengthened through development of criteria at each level which might subsequently evolve into a theoretical framework of thrownness.

Death and dying

At a higher level of severity in the taxonomy of thrownness it was evident that students felt vulnerable in a personal and professional way. Being unprepared in situations of great importance such as counselling bereaved relatives and dealing with terminally ill patients/clients can feel extremely threatening to the inexperienced nurse [whether a student or not]. There appears to be an expectation that students will be able to cope, even though it is likely that they will have received little, if any, supervision or teaching about such situations. Conflict occurs between personal and professional Selves and emotional and cognitive areas of action. Macleod Clark et al. (1996) and I provide evidence that students are still expected to learn through doing and they do not always have the opportunity to observe the skills which they need to acquire. This is an extremely important issue because it is likely that, due to the sensitive nature of counselling and caring for dying patients, students may not be exposed to experts in action in such situations. It is therefore imperative that scenarios are created in a safe learning environment in which students can explore the topic and their own emotions in relation to death and dying and to learn possible lines of action and response. As students may be confronted by death on their first day in nursing practice it may be very worthwhile to include sessions on death and dying very early in the nurse education programme. Qualified nurses acting as supervisors need to recognise levels of support required by each individual student. Rescue strategies might be explored during clinical supervision for instance, or simply as part of the care administered for particular patients/clients on an everyday basis. Within my study, students demonstrated personal investment of Self in situations dealing with death, dying and bereavement. To some extent, responding to such situations can be taught and learned, but many actions and responses depend upon the intuitive nature of the individual. Educationalists might consider how this type of intuition can be fostered and developed through experiential and reflective approaches to education.

Whilst The Peach Report (UKCC, 1999; 5.27) identifies that students require more adequate preparation for practice placements in order to be able to function safely and effectively, my study has taken this issue further by identifying a particular area of nursing practice which requires immediate attention. It appears that, in the past, curriculum planners have delayed formal tuition in relation to death and dying to the later stages of the Course, believing that students might be responsible for dealing with it from a managerial perspective. It is evident, however, that students need to be equipped with the basic skills to protect themselves from threat as, say, they would in protecting themselves from back pain from lifting.

Supervision of students in clinical practice

Recognition that the healthcare environment has been under pressure for a long time, with more patients and fewer nursing staff, no shift overlaps and changes to delivery of care means that students often receive inconsistent, ineffectual and poor supervision in clinical practice. In addition to these major factors, participants in my study were allocated to placements for two or three days a week during the CFP, which was insufficient to develop relationships with supervisors and patients or to develop skills pertinent to the particular area of nursing. Whilst the participants in my study experienced varying

251

'models' of supervision, they perceived that relationships might be strengthened, given extended periods of time on a placement. The Peach Commission (UKCC, 1999; 4.42) recognised that short, poorly-planned placements can prevent students from developing even basic skills and students have been criticised for not being 'streetwise' because they are often unused to working shift patterns, working within the multidisciplinary team or dealing with difficult situations. The implication is that students might benefit from longer placements throughout the Diploma course.

My student participants experienced and portrayed examples of 'good' and 'poor' supervisory practice and described the desirable traits of good supervisors [Chapter 8]. Most of them identified experiences of effective supervision which enabled them to explore aspects of nursing practice, such as teaching and management, in a safe, reassuring and encouraging learning environment. Students valued time to reflect upon their practice with their supervisors and self-assessment appears to be a healthy way of identifying professional development needs. Damage caused to students through expectations based on assumption of a single progression through the Course cannot be underestimated. At the time of this study students experienced different placements and there was no standard trajectory through the Course. Because of this, students had difficulty in transferring skills learned on one placement to others. It appears that learning in some placements was context bound. It is therefore, imperative that supervisors, rather than assuming students' existing knowledge because of their stage of progression through the Course, spend some time with the student discussing learning which has occurred in previous placements. Students would benefit from interviews with their supervisors at the earliest possible opportunity.

Good supervision was also instrumental in whether students were accepted by nursing and multidisciplinary teams, as was demonstrated in the Present Tense Commentaries. This feeling of integration, particularly in the Branch Programmes, helped students to develop a professional self-image which gave them more confidence to make a contribution in practice. Self-actualisation and the desire for personal and professional growth are inextricably linked and is seems that if basic needs are met, students strive to fulfil their potential within the team.

My study participants developed an awareness and understanding for various aspects of nursing at different stages of the Course. There is no evidence to suggest that they all developed the same skills at the same time which previous nurse socialisation studies have implied (Bradby, 1989; Day et al. 1995; Macleod Clark et al. 1996; Melia, 1981; Philpin, 1999). Each individual, depending upon their experience, maturity, interest in the placement and standard of supervision, learned and developed differently. However, it is evident from my study that students need to make sense of their situations before they can become active subjects. There is the danger that, if the environment is not conducive to students' development, they may become an active subject, but at an inappropriate (i.e. auxiliary) level.

Using hermeneutic phenomenology

To satisfy the aims of the study, I strove for a research strategy and philosophical and theoretical frameworks which enabled a thorough exploration of issues raised by my student participants and which also permitted me to contribute to the data as a participant. Heidegger's work, "Being and Time" attracted my interest because of its focus on care and concern and because I could draw parallels between his hermeneutic phenomenology and my own experiences within nursing and nurse education. His arguments and claims seemed especially germane to nursing and I subsequently endeavoured to adhere to the underlying philosophical stance during the research process. The philosophical and methodological choices I made for this study evolved from my belief that the art and science of nursing should evolve from an ontological base.

The traditional frameworks and theories used by many earlier researchers in nursing (Henderson, 1960; Johnson, 1980; King, 1971; Orem, 1980; Roper, Logan and Tierney, 1985) view human wholeness as made up of a combination of physiological, psychological and spiritual attributes, which are studied separately and then placed together as a whole entity. More recent authors/theorists acknowledge the relevance of hermeneutic phenomenology to nursing (Annells, 1996; Munhall, 1994; Parse, 1992; Taylor, 1994). The theoretical structures of Parse's (1981) theory of human becoming, for example, are indicative of the way that nursing is moving toward an understanding of the meaning of lived experience.

A further rationale for choosing this approach included a need to be 'in there' myself, as I believed that I could not be objective in my descriptions of students' experiences or utilise an approach which advocates 'bracketing' (Husserl, 1962). Hermeneutic phenomenology emphasises valuing individuals' personal structures of their lifeworld; co-creating reality; acknowledging that meaning continuously changes as experiences create new understandings; interacting and connecting with other people to co-constitute meaning and believing that 'becoming' is an open process differently experienced by each person. Working within these principles enabled the purpose of the approach to be realised, that is, I uncovered the structure of lived experience with students who articulated the meaning they assigned to it.

The benefits of using a hermeneutic approach for this study include; an emphasis upon students' stories rather than a researcher agenda; lived experience being seen to precede understanding; the multiple perspective of temporality; deepening and broadening of understandings through a fusion of horizons; an appreciation for unique and diverse experiences and meanings; the provision of multiple interpretations of the phenomenon and the seeing of new ways of being. For me, the single most difficult aspect of satisfying a hermeneutic approach was the demand for congruency within all activities associated with the research process. If one makes an uninformed decision with regard to data collection or analysis for example, it may result in a poor fit between method/technique and philosophical principles. Such dissonance was experienced by Koch (1994), who had to radically alter Colaizzi's (1978) analysis framework, because it was not congruent with the Heideggerian and Gadamerian principles she was using.

Using hermeneutic phenomenology has taught me a self-discipline which I might not have acquired using other approaches. Attempting to fulfil the demands of the hermeneutic circle often led to an unprecedented thoroughness which, on occasions, tried my patience and consumed a great deal of time. The hermeneutic circle is difficult to initiate and maintain and nursing research which claims to use hermeneutics is testimony to this difficulty (Annells, 1996; Moustakas, 1994; Packer and Addison, 1989; van Manen, 1990). Despite the demands of a hermeneutic approach, it is thoroughly congruent with the nature and discipline of nursing and nurse education.

Theoretical and philosophical harmony? An evaluation

Although Ashworth (1981) discusses alliances between phenomenology and Kelly's Personal Construct Theory, my study appears to be unique as a working example of how the theories complement each other from both philosophical and pragmatic perspectives. I am also unaware of any other studies within the nurse education literature which make comparisons of the concept of the person from both phenomenological and constructivist viewpoints.

Many phenomenologists emphasise the importance of analysis being concerned with 'primordial phenomena' (Kockelmans, 1967, p29), "phenomena in their unmediated and originary manifestation to consciousness" (Natanson, 1974, p8), "phenomena presenting themselves in immediate experience" (Pickles, 1985, p178), supporting the view that experience should not be subjected to self-conscious rational processes. But I argue that stories of experience cannot be conveyed to another person without some reflection or attempts to understand the effects of the experience. No-one can access another's experience if the first party is not aware of it themself. Also, if the researcher is to understand lifeworld through an interpretation of data, then the researcher's interpretation of the participant's lifeworld will be more in accord with the primary experiencer if the participant has reflected upon their experiences first.

Using original methods and techniques

I made decisions about the methodology as the study progressed. At times this somewhat unpredictable way of progressing was unnerving, but it provided flexibility and responsiveness to participants' needs.

Researchers who have used Personal Construct Theory and Repertory Grid Technique in nursing and nurse education (Barnes, 1990; Buckenham, 1998; Heyman, Shaw and Harding, 1983; Morrison, 1990; Pollock, 1986; Scholes and Freeman, 1994) have tended to do so on a one-off basis, without supplementary data sources and to study students at a single point in time which gives little insight into the changing nature of their participants' constructs.

Buckenham (1998) argues that Kellyan RepGrid should be used several times with the same individual over a period of time enabling an analysis of changing constructs during the education process. If the intention is to monitor and measure changing constructs using statistics, then repeated use of the technique would serve the purpose. As I wanted to understand the meaning that students assigned to their changing constructs, RepGrid as the single data collection technique was not enough. The evolutionary nature of my data collection strategy meant that I was able to ask students themselves about their construing and how constructions evolved. To me, this was a far more interesting, worthwhile and fruitful path of enquiry. The way I developed the use of the grids meant that students could ignore and omit aspects of the grid which they felt had no current meaning for them. This gave me insight into their changing constructs, sometimes without any verbal explanation. Using an evolutionary scheme to collect material provided the desired insight into students' constructs. In Chapter 6, I used Kelly's

Personal Construct Theory more readily than hermeneutics as a framework to discuss issues associated with 'intentionality' because the material was concerned with perceptions, anticipations and expectations of nursing and the education programme, that is, the students' constructs were accessible as perception or opinion and not as experience per se. This meant that I could make more sense of the data using a constructivist perspective than a phenomenological one. This material served as a baseline for the subsequent chapters such as 'experiences of thrownness' and 'being-in-the-world-with-others' where hermeneutics was a more suitable framework for illuminating students' experience. I used a modified repertory grid for the third data collection phase which took the form of a reflective dialogue that enabled students to relate current issues in the context of past understandings. This was achieved because I used the students' own statements from earlier one-to-one interviews. The use of elements from the students' own dialogue in my study meant that students could identify the stimuli of change, examine their current situation in the light of new learning and attribute meaning to the process as a whole. This is an original approach to using the grid in the context of studies of nursing and contrasts with Morrison's (1991) use of the technique whereby he selected elements upon which his students commented.

Developing the Present Tense Commentary technique, from an original idea by Witkin (1994), proved to be rewarding as it provided a privileged insight into the students' lifeworld because I was involved in the story as it was told. Witkin's ideas were extended by including reflection and using the student's own material from data gathered earlier. I would argue that this is a significant contribution to developing a reflective scheme which might assist students to analyse their practice more fully. Present Tense Commentary might be a useful technique within a clinical/supervisory relationship to facilitate reflection-on-action, providing that individuals are emotionally protected as I suggest in Chapter 3. There is potential to develop my existing work with this technique (Mitchell, 1999) and I expect to invite collaboration in an empirical study to explore and evaluate Present Tense Commentary as a tool to recall practice situations, with the aim of enhancing qualified and student nurses' professional development. This would complement the recommendation made in the Peach Report (UKCC, 1999; 4.23), that all practice-based learning should be assessed through portfolios of practice experience which would highlight any deficits in the students' development, so that remedial action can be taken.

Using students' Reflective Practice Portfolios and Letter Writing as material for my study extends the existing work on aesthetic knowing in nursing (Carper, 1978; Vezeau, 1993; Appleton, 1991). I am not aware of any other nursing studies using letter writing as a method in research and hope that doing so might fuel discussion regarding the use of more creative means for gaining access to the experiences of health care personnel and patients/clients. The letters from my participants provided insight into other aspects of their lifeworlds apart from the professional perspective which was especially valuable in creating the introductory and concluding prose in Part IV. I intend to write for general consumption about letter writing as a source of research material.

Commitment to data analysis

Chapter 3 described how I considered and rejected various formal analysis frameworks (e.g. Colaizzi, 1978; Giorgi, 1985) on the grounds that they are more specifically suited to phenomenological psychology studies than to hermeneutic studies.

Commitment to the hermeneutic circle is evident in my decision to use both formal and informal analysis frameworks to detect similarities and uniqueness within the students' accounts. This activity was essential for me to identify individual meanings of common experiences and common meanings of individual experiences. Weaving in and out of each data set for an individual and through a single data set for all individuals facilitated my understanding of issues on a micro and macro level of abstraction. Enrolling colleagues to discuss emerging issues from the material assisted and broadened my perspective in relation to individual students' experiences and I would advise using this activity to share experiences in order to clarify thoughts. I gave my colleagues a clear remit which did not include verification of students' experiences or my interpretations of them, but more simply, to indicate whether they themselves could recognise the experiences and my interpretation. This appears to be an original approach in the nursing and nurse education literature.

Willingness to acknowledge emerging Selves

Another example of personal discipline using hermeneutics is the continual examination of Self as researcher and as the main research tool. I found the challenge of recognising my multiple Selves within the research process enlightening while reflecting upon the processes

257

involved in the research overwhelmed me at times with a feeling of insecurity, naivety and unpreparedness. My own development was not always obvious, although the ability to be thorough and make considered decisions based upon experience and knowledge became more recognisable as I gained experience as a researcher. In the early stages of the research I found difficulty with the freedom of reflexivity which allowed me to choose personally relevant issues for the research, draw on and make explicit personal experience and enjoy the wisdom and companionship of the research participants (Bannister, 1981).

Part of the insight gained into my professional Selves occurred through scrutinising transcript texts, but in the main, the realisation occurred through listening to my own voice on tape [interviews and dictaphone recording of my diary]. When using an interpretive scheme such as Heideggerian hermeneutics, attention to discourse and articulation are essential if understanding by the researcher is to be achieved. At the outset of this study I was aware of the importance of listening to my participants, but interest in my own development was gradual and took me some time to realise. The importance of my emerging Selves and the influence these have had on the study have been framed as part of the context of the study.

It seems appropriate that the final section of my thesis relates to the use of reflection as part of the research strategy and as a tool which raised my own awareness about personal and professional influences upon the study. The concept of reflective practice in nursing and nurse education has increased in popularity because of its potential to connect theory with practice, knowing with doing and personal with professional development. Although reflection is fundamentally epistemological, reflection-on-action and in-action is ontological because it enables 'being' to be elucidated and analysed and is therefore, congruent with all aspects of this study.

The student's reflecting-on-action

Reflective practice was a new concept to my participants when I first introduced it during the RepGrid encounters. Several students found difficulty in completing their grids fully because they were unable to forecast how they might construe situations as a qualified nurse. More pertinently, they experienced some difficulty with reflecting on perceptions at the outset of the Course because of problems of relevance; that is, they could not always remember why they had made some of the comments at the beginning of the Course, as they assigned

258

no current meaning to them. In some ways, this enabled them to see their progression which they found particularly rewarding.

The guidelines I produced for students to prepare for the Present Tense Commentaries were said to be useful in assisting with the method and in making sense of subsequent experiences in nursing practice at a later date.

The value of the Reflective Practice Portfolios was acknowledged by students as an opportunity to examine and assess their performance, identify problems and comment on what had occurred. Using the portfolios as material for this study provided additional insight into their reflections which made my interpretation of events more rounded. These reflections gave me the advantage of seeing their experiences through their lenses of perception which contributed to my perceptions of their lifeworld.

Students reported that reflection had been an 'enlightening experience', useful for identifying how feelings and emotions were provoked, for personal progress and what was yet to be learned. They all reported that reflection was useful as a practical tool and could see the potential benefit of it to their professional development and to patient care. The creation of knowledge through the transformation of experience and knowing about practice enabled students to make decisions, problem-solve and interject in practice situations which, in turn, made them feel valued. This change in capability through knowledge and skill acquisition led to greater autonomy and this is evidenced in the experiences which have been framed as 'active subject' [Chapter 10].

My reflections-on-action

I reflected upon all the methods I used in order to promote my understanding and keep information context bound in accordance with a hermeneutic approach. I tried to stand back to observe why things were either going well or not so well. This might seem somewhat paradoxical when I have argued that 'bracketing' was not achievable. By 'standing back' I mean that I took time from what I was doing to consider past actions and how they were fashioned in the light of my limited experience.

One of the purposes of using reflection for some of the data collection phases was to achieve a 'convergence of meaning' between myself and the students so that I might understand their perspective. I found that the data collection strategies which depended upon reflection-on-action worked because the students and I shared a frame of reference rooted in nursing practice, shared language, contexts and processes. This was necessary as part of the hermeneutic circle where meaning and understanding evolved through weaving in and out of data, experiences, frames of reference and interpretations. The term 'responsive choreography' (Davis and Sumara, 1997) is appropriate to describe the importance of this convergence through a reciprocal arrangement of mutual understanding and respect.

I consider that the ability to reflect depends upon the individual's ability to remember, recall, describe, relive, view from different perspectives, have an empathy with others of a different opinion and be able to recognise potential learning opportunities. It is understandable therefore, that students' reflective skills took some time to develop, but that substantial improvements are evident between their efforts to reflect at the beginning and then the later stages of the research. Reflection can be difficult for those who have a poor capacity to remember. I acknowledged the fallibility of memory and provided students with guidelines and prompts for the methods and techniques which required them to reflect.

Through reflexivity my inappropriate decisions during the research process were modified and new approaches were sought in which new ideas and possibilities were expounded, for example, with regard to using RepGrids, Present Tense Commentary and Letter Writing. Without such recording, the study may have been quite different - adhering to more traditional interview methods, rather than taking risks with new ones. I reflected upon my own historicity to determine whether my experience would be more useful in some methods rather than in others and reflected upon my standard of communication skills, how I used humour, how students might feel in certain situations and how they had already reacted to me during previous data collection phases.

There is an obligation, using hermeneutics, for the researcher to reflect on pre-understandings and how these develop through continued reading, writing and interpretation. Although I have attempted to situate myself within the study, I think I could have provided more insight for the reader into my pre-understandings in relation to my views about Project 2000. I regret finding Geanellos' (1998) work too late for it to influence this study, but there is scope for me to take her work on board for future projects. She emphasises the imperative of examining fore-understandings more thoroughly and explicitly as part of a hermeneutic approach and demonstrates her own process of doing so in her research. Her process is documented well and would be useful as a guide if I use diary and critical incident material with Present Tense Commentary in the future project mentioned earlier. This process would enable fore-understandings to be brought to consciousness in order to provide the phenomenon under investigation with the greatest opportunity to reveal itself (Geanellos, 1998, p238). Like Geanellos, I could have generated statements about my forestructures and then reconceptualised them in the light of my findings. This process would have enabled a more thorough exposure of my beliefs and biases within this study.

Finally, I had to make decisions about what was included in the original thesis which also required a reflective approach to analysis and selection of relevant experiences. The students' stories, of course, are incomplete because of word constraints for the thesis. There is as much, if not more, material remaining than I used in the thesis and I share the sentiment of Lofland and Lofland (1984) who describe the 'agony of omitting' many of the students' stories from this, the written product of the research. I expect to be able to use the remaining material in various presentations; within my teaching, during seminars and in publications.

Very recently the Faculty in which I work has been selected as one of sixteen sites to pilot the recommendations of The Peach Report. I am looking forward with interest to being involved in the planning and implementation of the recommendations and to contributing findings and experiences from my own study. My main hope in conducting the research and writing the thesis is that it resonates with others to provide a source of interest, discussion and action for the benefit of nursing and nurse education.

Appendices

Appendices

1 Kelly's (1955) Fundamental Postulate and Eleven Corollaries

Fundamental postulate

"A person's processes are psychologically channelized by the ways he [sic] anticipates events."

The corollaries

Construction corollary

"A person anticipates events by construing their replications."

Individuality corollary

"Persons differ from each other in their construction of events."

Organisation corollary

"Each person characteristically evolves, for his convenience in anticipating events, a construction system embracing ordinal relationships between constructs."

Dichotomy corollary

"A person's construction system is composed of a finite number of dichotomous constructs."

Choice corollary

"A person chooses for himself [sic] that alternative in a dichotomised construct through which he anticipates the greater possibility for extension and definition of his system."

Range corollary

"A construct is convenient for the anticipation of a finite range of events only."

Experience corollary

"A person's construction system varies as he successively construes the replications of events."

Modulation corollary

"The variation in a person's construction is limited by the permeability of the constructs within range of convenience the variants lie."

Fragmentation corollary

"A person may successively employ a variety of construction subsystems which is similar to that employed by another, his psychological processes are similar to those of the other person."

Commonality corollary

"To the extent that one person employs a construction of experience which is similar to that employed by another, his psychological processes are similar to those of the other person."

Sociality corollary

"To the extent that one person construes the construction processes of another, he [sic] may play a role in a social process involving the other person."

2 Student Questionnaire, February 1994

Name:

1. Why do you want to be a nurse?

2. What do you know about the Course?

3. What qualifications, skills or personal characteristics do you have, which might help you on the Course?

4. What do you think are the characteristics of a 'good' nurse?

3 Interview Guide - Student Nurses

Tell me a bit about yourself and what you were doing prior to the Course commencing.

Do you have any nursing experience?

Did you have any anxieties prior to starting the Course?

What influenced your decision to become a nurse?

What were your expectations of the Course?

What are the qualities of a 'good nurse?

Have you encountered any difficulties as a student nurse?

How do you feel you fit into the group?

How do you feel you fit into nursing?

Have you changed as a result of completing six months on the Course?

4 Guidelines for Present Tense Commentary

This data collection technique is quite different to the interview and grid we used before.

The idea is for you to tell me about 2 events which have been significant to you during the Course so far. You can choose whether they are practice or college related, or one of each. One situation should be associated with an issue from list A and one from list B.

List A	List B
A situation which was familiar and comfortable for you	A situation where you felt uncomfortable in an unfamiliar environment
A situation where you really had a sense of belonging	A situation where you felt totally rejected
A situation where your values were in harmony with your actions	A situation where your values were in conflict with your actions
A situation where you felt confident	A situation where you felt unsure
A situation where you felt competent	A situation where you felt incompetent

Choose the incident carefully. To help you recall the incident, it might be helpful to use the questions for structured reflection on the attached page. Answer the question in as much detail as possible as this will help you to recall the incident and me to understand your perspective.

When we meet, you will be invited to describe the incident as if it is happening now - that is, in the present tense.

For example;

"I am sitting at my desk wondering what to write. I understand the meaning of the question, but am unable to think of the words to convey what I am feeling. This makes me feel anxious and I know it will add to the pressure when I do not achieve the deadline for my assignment. I'm going to make yet another cup of coffee to ponder my predicament. I have two options as I see it - I can contact my supervisor, or just write a substandard essay. I would feel guilty if I phoned my supervisor as it is the weekend. I feel desperate and inadequate. I can't do this."

It is quite difficult to talk through an incident in the present tense so I will help you maintain focus. I hope that reflecting first will help you to recall the detail and bring it forward to the present tense.

I look forward to meeting with you again. In the meantime, do not hesitate to contact me if you have any problems.

Regards

Theresa Mitchell

Telephone (Work):

Telephone (Home):

Appointment date for discussion and problem-solving

Commentary meeting date –

5 Model for Structured Reflection (Johns, 1995; Carper, 1978)

1. Describe the experience:

2. What factors contributed to this experience?

3. Who are the actors in the experience?

4. Why did you do what you did?

5. How did you feel whilst this was happening?

6. What factors influenced your decision?

7. What were the consequences of your actions?

8. Could you have dealt better with the situation?

9. What other choices did you have?

10. How did you feel about the experience?

11. How has the experience changed your practice?

6 End of Course Questionnaire

Name:

1. Explain what you understood about nursing prior to the Course.

   Was this an accurate perception?

2. Briefly, how have you developed personally during the Course?

3. Briefly, how have you developed professionally during the Course?

4. At what stage, if at all, did you feel that you belonged to the nursing profession?

5. What factors contributed to you completing the Course?

6. If you were selecting potential nursing students, how would you select them?

7. What particular events during the Course, have been significant to your development?

8. What factors determined whether you felt accepted into nursing?

9. Did you ever feel like giving up? At what stage did this occur?

10. How do you feel about becoming a staff nurse?

11. What are you looking forward to as a qualified nurse?

Thankyou for your co-operation.

7 Guidelines for Letter Writing

To conclude the data collection for my study, I would be very grateful if you would write a detailed letter to an imaginary friend/relative whom you have not seen for several years.

It is the intention of the letter to summarise your personal and professional development during the last three years, in becoming a nurse. The letter will provide some insight into the experiences to which you assign the greatest importance and aspects of clinical practice and education which have influenced your development.

Perhaps you might include the following:

- The impetus for choosing nursing as a career
- Supporting networks/individuals
- Motivations to continue
- Events which made you feel elated
- Events which made you feel miserable
- Future ambitions, hopes and fears

I am indebted to you for your continued co-operation. As in previous data collection phases, I respect your right to confidentiality.

Many thanks.

8 Reinharz's (1983) Analysis Framework

1. Participants transform their private experiences into language which is taped and transcribed, leaving a large space on the right hand side for written interpretations.

2. Repeated and careful listening of the experiences and reflections upon them to gain a general idea of the meaning of these experiences. As you listen, visualise the conversations with the participants so that their emotional state is noted and interpretations become more personal. Re-read and reflect upon the transcripts several times over a period of weeks.

3. This understanding is then transformed into conceptual themes which capture the essence of each participants' experience. The themes will emerge from a dialectic process of moving between a background of intersubjective or shared meanings and one of focused meanings specific to the participants' experience. This is the hermeneutic circle. As the researcher's interpretations become clearer, similar themes may merge into larger essential themes.

4. The essential themes are then transformed into a meaningful written document that enables new understandings to be publicly expressed.

5. The final process of understanding is performed by the reader, when interpretations are created out of the experiences of the participants.

9 The Six Most Relevant Corollaries Used to Interpret Data

The individuality corollary

This corollary provides grounds for individual difference in the anticipation of events. Through construing events or situations, an individual moves towards an interpretation of their world.

I used this corollary to organise the raw data which had personal meaning for students. Personal perceptions of the Course, family support, personal abilities and students' constructions of their relationships were assigned to this corollary.

Much of this data comprises 'I' statements where it is obvious that the student owns what has been said and does not seek common ground with their counterparts. Kelly (1991) perceives that individuals can be found living out their existence next door to each other, but in different subjective worlds. Some of the statements could be easily shared with other students, but at the time that it was said, no connections were made with others.

The individuality corollary does not mean that there can be no sharing of experiences. Whilst there may be many individual constructions of events in which the student is involved, it does not mean that these constructions are divorced from anothers constructions of the same event.

The commonality corollary

This corollary implies that there is similarity in the construction of events between individuals. Kelly (op. cit.) believes that, taken from a phenomenological perspective, no two persons can have either the same construction, or the same psychological processes.

This would make the commonality corollary unrealistic. The only possibility in this instance is that two people's psychological processes

276

may be construed as similar.

Having trawled the students' raw data, it became apparent that they became anxious about similar events. One of these events was the nature of academic assignments and how the results of the assignment caused particular distress. Another common construct to all 'adult general' nursing students was the need to develop an identity.

I also included data associated with perceived lack of practical skills taught on the Course in this corollary. In relation to this, they construed their world as being more student oriented than nurse oriented.

Kelly states that certain groups of people behave similarly in certain respects. Some of these similarities are associated with age, some may be in relation to experience and some related with other constructions of similarity.

The sociality corollary

While a common or similar cultural background tends to make people see things alike, it does not guarantee cultural progress. It does not even guarantee social harmony. This corollary enabled me to identify the extent that one person construed the construction processes of another, so that they could play a role in a social process which involved other persons. I believed this to be particularly pertinent to statements associated with students' perceptions of clinical colleagues and how they felt they were fitting into clinical nursing practice. It also had an application in relation to role models and how they affected students' development. In the main, statements demonstrated an appreciation of other nursing roles, ability to relate to the role of the qualified nurse, attitudes towards trained staff and how uniform provided a status which enabled students to belong to the nursing culture.

Kelly states that if we can predict accurately what others will do, we can adjust ourselves to their behaviour. This can be seen in some of the statements I categorised within this corollary about how one student described how she believed that students should be seen to be 'good' which endears them to their qualified colleagues. Kelly defines 'role' as an ongoing pattern of behaviour that follows from the person's understanding of how others who are associated with him in the task, think. In short, a role is a position that one can play on a certain team without even waiting for their signals. it is the students' desire for a 'place' within nursing that is most evident in this data.

The experience corollary

The succession of events in the course of time continually subjects a person's construct system to a validation process. The constructions one places upon events are working hypotheses which are about to be put to the test of experience. These hypotheses are successively revised in the light of unfolding events and the construction undergoes a progressive evolution. The reconstruction of one's life is based upon this kind of experience and it may reshape the person's system by stabilising or disrupting the original construct. In the experience corollary, construing may be seen as a series of events along a path of time. Within this corollary, I included statements about past experiences which the students brought forward and in response, modified their constructs or raised awareness. Kelly's explanation of this corollary appears to be similar to reflection-on-action and comprises examination of past experience and the lifting of valuable discoveries to enrich the meaning of present and future experiences.

Within this corollary, I assigned raw data associated with changing attitudes and evidence of students' construing events based on their previous experience. The set of data contained within this corollary includes examples of students change in attitude, changes in perceptions of the Course and personal and professional change.

The dichotomy corollary

In Kelly's theory, it is recognised that a person anticipates events by noting their replicative aspects. By the same token, they may also anticipate events by noting their contrasting aspects. Kelly describes the dichotomy corollary in terms associated with equations, which appeared cumbersome, I preferred to use it to contrast constructs held by the same individual. Constructs can structure a person's thinking and can limit their access to the ideas of others.

Within this corollary I categorised statements which demonstrated some cognitive incongruency between constructs held by an individual. Sometimes the contrasting stimuli produced through observation and the students own construing of events, threw the individual into turmoil. They did not know what to believe and sometimes their thought became irrational. There is also evidence of confusion within these statements which, I think, shows how dichotomous some of the contrasting constructs can be. There is also evidence of contrast between what is expected and what is real.

The fragmentation corollary

A person's construction system is continually in a state of flux, however, new constructs are not necessarily derivatives of old constructs. The old and new constructs may be incompatible with each other. Kelly discusses fragmentation as opposite to consistency, but that consistency relates to the successive use of subsystems which, in themselves, do not add up. Within this corollary, I considered statements which students offered related to perceived inconsistencies in the Course content, in expectations of the Course and events which required a quick shift of personal attitude or role. Kelly acknowledges that this quick turn around of construing events can lead a person to anticipate reality in bizarre ways.

The issues addressed within this corollary relate to the inconsistency between two constructs such as home and nursing life. Also, the difference between constructions of nursing.

10 An Example of a Discussion with Colleagues as Part of the Analysis Strategy

A brief summary of the meeting;-

Both colleagues commented that they understood, and could relate to, the concept of thrownness. This understanding was brought about through their experiences as tutors and nurses and through their observations of students being 'thrown'.

Richard had some trouble coming to terms with the structure and style of the chapter and sought clarification of some terms. Alison, who had been reading literature on phenomenology, felt more comfortable with the structure and style. Interestingly, they both enjoyed my interpretation of personal and professional Selves and how I described the merging of these in some instances evident in the students' data. Their interest may mean that this is an area for further consideration and development.

I used the term 'dumped' in the chapter to describe the experience of one student who had been ill-prepared to cope with a particular situation and Richard tended to think that this was rather a colloquial term. Alison liked it and said that she believed that the term described exactly what she had experienced as a student and has subsequently observed as a tutor. Richard commented that his dislike of the term may stem from a desire to defend his role as a tutor; he knew that students should not be 'dumped' and felt some responsibility for this happening in clinical practice.

We had considerable discussion relating to students exposure to death and dying in nursing practice and Richard felt that I had made a few sweeping statements which I will attend to. We reflected on our own experiences of nursing and remembered how difficult it could be.

Richard suggested that a degree of reverence and an appropriate attitude whilst dealing with dying patients and bereaved relatives might possibly help relieve nurses' anxiety and may, in itself, be a rescue strategy.

Both Richard and Alison agreed that the professional Self strengthens as students progress through the Course, but they recognised the 'sink or swim' mentality which still prevails in nursing practice.

Richard's story of thrownness involved students expectation of nursing in the accident and emergency department in comparison with the television programme, 'E R'. Perceptively, Richard talked about how, on television, the camera enjoys the richness of each scenario happening behind curtains and how the viewer is informed from an all-observing, all-knowing perspective. In real life, one nurse is most often assigned to one patient and therefore does not have insight into all cases behind the curtains. Richard believed that students are thrown by this restricted perspective and that they are disappointed that their experience in the department is not as exciting as anticipated.

Alison's story of thrownness occurred during her teaching of "candidates" for life support training (interesting that she calls these learners candidates and not students). She stated that she noticed a conflict between personal and professional Selves in these learners and compared this to her own experience as an intensive care nurse when she was out with the paramedics. She remembered being called out to a relatively minor accident but found herself in a state of thrownness because she did not have all the usual equipment in the intensive care unit, available to her. She said that she was almost paralysed because she could not improvise and she did not know what to do. She reported that in a different context, she would have been competent to manage such a situation, but was thrown by the unfamiliar environment of Park Lane and lack of equipment.

I concluded the meeting by summarising the main points of the chapter and clarifying how I perceived they had understood, and related to, the content.

11 Themes Generated from Focus Groups with Tutors

Mature students
Media influence
Role models
Academic support
Student motivation
Previous nursing experience
Student perceptions of nursing
Academic ability
Student nurse - Nursing student
Expectations
'Bad' nurse characteristics
Teacher influences
Life experience
Preparation for practice
Inappropriate career choice
Selection methods
Qualifications
Students with degrees
Changing role of the tutor
Relationships
Social/personal problems
The product
Satisfying a need
Course culture
Theory/practice
Course organisation
Identity and belonging
Uniform
Tutors in clinical practice
Clinical staff influences
Ideas for student selection

12 Themes Generated from Interviews with Practitioners

The supervisory role
Role models
Traditional Versus Project 2000 students
Practical skills
Supervisor as facilitator
Pleasantly surprised
Supervisor/student relationship
A different type of student
Feeling equal - professional threat to qualified staff
Perceptions of the Course
Understanding students' needs
Students' problems
Expectations of students
Undesirable characteristics of student nurses

References

References

Akerlind, G.S., Jenkins, S. (1998) Academic's views of the relative roles and responsibilities of teachers and learners in a first year university course, *Higher Education Research and Development*, Vol. 17, No. 3, pp277-288.

Alavi, C., Cooke, M., Crowe, M. (1997) Becoming a registered nurse, *Nurse Education Today*, Vol. 7, pp473-480.

Alcoff, L. (1988) Cultural feminism versus post structuralism? Identity crisis in feminist theory, *Signs*, Vol. 13, No. 3, pp405-436.

Allen, M.N., Jenson, L. (1990) Hermeneutic enquiry: Meaning and scope, *Western Journal of Nursing Research*, Vol. 12, pp241-253.

Anderson, L.E. (1994) A new look at an old construct: Cross-cultural adaptation, *International Journal of Intercultural Relations*, Vol. 18, pp293-328.

Anderson, R.J., Hughes, J.A., Sharrock, W.W. (1998) *Philosophy and the Human Sciences*, Croomhelm, Beckenham, Kent.

Annells, M. (1996) Hermeneutic phenomenology: philosophical perspectives and current use in nursing research, *Journal of Advanced Nursing*, Vol. 23, pp705-713.

Appleton, C.D. (1991) *The Gift of Self: The Meaning of the Art of Nursing*, University Microfilms International, 1992.

Appleton, J.V. (1995) Analysing qualitative interview data: addressing issues of validity and reliability, *Journal of Advanced Nursing*, Vol. 22, pp993-997.

Ashcroft, K., Foreman-Peck, L. (1994) *Managing Teaching and Learning in Further and Higher Education*, The Falmer Press, London.

Ashton, H., Shuldham, C. (1994) An exploratory study of students' perceptions of the benefits of regular small group tutorials in a 2 year day-release course, *Journal of Advanced Nursing*, Vol. 20, pp925-934.

Ashworth, P.D. (1981) Equivocal alliances of phenomenological psychology, *Journal of Phenomenological Psychology*, Vol. 12, No. 1, pp1-31.

Ashworth, P.D. (1986) (ed) *Qualitative Research in Psychology*, Duquesne University Press, Pittsburgh, Pennsylvania.

Bailey, C.A. (1996) *A Guide to Field Research*, Pine Forge Press, Thousand Oaks, CA.

Bailie, R., Steinberg, M. (1995) The focus group method in a formative evaluation of a South African high school sexuality education programme, *The British Journal of Family Planning*, Vol. 21, pp71-75.

Bannister, D. (1981) Personal construct theory and research method, Chapter 16, in Reason, P., Rowan, J. (eds), *Human Inquiry*, John Wiley and Sons Ltd, New York.

Bannister, D., Fransella, F. (1986) *Inquiring Man: The Psychology of Personal Constructs*, 3rd edition, Croomhelm, London.

Bannister, D., Fransella, F., Agnew, J. (1971) Characteristics and validity of the grid test of thought disorder, *British Journal of Social and Clinical Psychology*, Vol. 10, pp144-151.

Banonis, B.C. (1989) The lived experience of recovering from addiction: A phenomenological study, *Nursing Research*, Vol. 41, No. 3, pp166-170.

Barker, M., Child, C., Gallois, C., Jones, E., Callan, V.J. (1991) Differences of overseas students in social and academic situations, *Australian Journal of Psychology*, Vol. 43, pp79-84.

Barnes, E. (1990) An examination of nurses' feelings about patients with specific feeding needs. *Journal of Advanced Nursing*, Vol. 15, pp703-711.

Beck, C.T. (1991) How students perceive faculty caring: A phenomenological study, *Nurse Educator*, Vol. 16, No. 5, Sept/Oct, pp19-22.

Beck, C.T. (1994) (1) Phenomenology: its use in nursing research, *International Journal of Nursing Studies*, Vol. 31, No. 6, pp499-510.

Beck, C.T. (1994) (2) Reliability and validity issues in phenomenological research, *Western Journal of Nursing Research*, Vol. 16, No. 3, pp254-267.

Becker, C.S. (1992) *Living and Relating: An Introduction to Phenomenology*, Sage Publications, Newbury Park, London, New Delhi, pp25-28.

Becker, H.S., Geer, B., Hughes, E.C. (1968) *Making the Grade*, Wiley, New York.

Becker, H.S., Geer, B., Hughes, E.C., Strauss, A.L. (1961) *Boys in White*, University of Chicago Press.

Beech, I. (1999) Bracketing in phenomenological research, *Nurse Researcher*, Vol. 6, No. 3, Spring, pp35-51.

Bendall, E. (1974) *The Relationship Between Recall and Application of Learning in Trainee Nurses*, Unpublished PhD thesis, London.

Benner, P. (1984) *From Novice to Expert. Experience and Power in Clinical Nursing Practice*, Addison Wesley, Menlo Park, California.

Benner, P., Wrubel, J. (1989) *The Primacy of Caring: Stress and Coping in Health and Illness*, Addison Wesley, Menlo-Park, California.

Benoliel, J.Q. (1977) The interaction between nursing theory and research, *Nursing Outlook*, Feb, Vol. 25, No. 2, pp108-113.

Bergum, V. (1991) Being a phenomenological researcher, in Morse, J. (ed), *Qualitative Nursing Research: A Contemporary Dialogue*, Sage Publications, Newbury Park, CA, pp55-71.

Berragan, L. (1997) Clinical Supervision: The implications for nursing, *Journal of Community Nursing*, Sept, Vol. 11, Issue 9, pp12-19.

Bleicher, J. (1980) *Contemporary Hermeneutics. Hermeneutics as Method, Philosophy and Critique*, Routledge and Kegan Paul, London.

Blumer, H. (1954) What is wrong with social theory? *American Sociological Review*, Vol. 19, pp3-10.

Blumer, H. (1969) *Symbolic Interactionism: Perspective and Method*, Prentice Hall, Englewood Cliffs, N.J.

Bobrow, D.G., Winograd, T. (1977) An overview of KRL, a knowledge representation language. *Cognitive Science*. Vol. 1, p32.

Bodley, D.E. (1991) Adapting supervision strategies to meet the challenges of future mental health nursing practice, *Nurse Education Today*, Vol. 11, pp378-386.

Bogdon, R., Taylor, S. (1984) *Introduction to Qualitative Reseach Methods*, 2nd Ed, Wiley Press, New York.

Bolton, N. (1979) Phenomenology and education, Unpublished inaugural lecture, cited in Ashworth, P.D. (1981) *Equivocal Alliances of Phenomenological Psychology*, Vol. 12, No. 1, pp1-31.

Bond, M. (1993) Older, wiser (and threatened), *Nursing Standard*, Vol. 7, No. 15, pp850-852.

Booth, K. (1992) Providing support and reducing stress: A review of the literature, in Butterworth, T., Faugier, J. (eds) *Clinical Supervision and Mentorship in Nursing*, Chapman and Hall, London.

288

Boud, D.J. (1991) Foreword in Hammond, M., Collins, R. *Self Directed Learning: Critical Practice*, Kogan Page, London.

Boud, D.J. (1995) *Enhancing Learning Through Self-Assessment*, Kogan Page, London.

Bowles, N. (1995) Methods of nurse selection: A review. *Nursing Standard*, Jan 4th, Vol. 9, No. 15, pp25-29.

Boyd, E., Fales, A. (1983) Reflective learning; key to learning from experience, *Journal of Humanistic Psychology*, Vol. 23, No. 2, pp99-117.

Boykin, A., Schoenhofer, S. (1991) Story as link between nursing practice, ontology and epistemology, Image *Journal of Nursing scholarship*, Vol. 23, No. 4, pp245-248.

Bradby, M.B. (1989) *Self Esteem and Status Passages: A Longitudinal Study of the Self-Perceptions of Nurses During Their First Year of Training*, Unpublished thesis, University of Exeter, Exeter.

Bradby, M.B. (1990) Status passage into nursing; another view of the process of socialization into nursing, *Journal of Advanced Nursing*, Oct 15th, Vol. 10, pp1220-1225.

Bradby, M., Soothill, K. (1993) From common foundation programme to branch: Recognising a status transition, *Nurse Education Today*, Vol. 13, No. 5, pp362-368.

Broadhead, R. (1983) *Private Lives and Professional Identity of Medical Students*, New Brunswick, Transaction, N.J.

Buckenham, M.A. (1998) Socialization and personal change: a personal construct theory approach, *Journal of Advanced Nursing*, Vol. 28, No. 4, pp874-881.

Burkitt, I. (1991) *Social Selves: Theories of Social Formation of Personality*, Sage Publications, London.

Burdett, P. (1998) *Supervision Needs of Student Nurses*, Unpublished M.Sc. dissertation, University of Bristol.

Burns, N. (1989) Standards for qualitative research, *Nursing Science Quarterly*, Spring, Vol. 1, pt. 1, pp44-52.

Burns, S. (1994) Assessing reflective learning, in Palarm, A., Burns, S., Bulman, C. (eds), *Reflective Practice in Nursing: The Growth of the Professional Practitioner*, Blackwell Science, Oxford.

Button, E. (1985) *Personal Construct Theory and Mental Health*, Croomhelm, London.

Cahill, H.A. (1996) A qualitative analysis of student nurses' experiences of mentorship, *Journal of Advanced Nursing*, 24, pp791-799.

Calder, B.J. (1977) Focus groups and the nature of qualitative marketing research. *Journal Marketing Research*, Vol. X1V, pp353-364.

Campbell, A.V. (1984) *Moderated love. A Theology of Professional Care*, Photobooks, Bristol.

Carper, B. (1978) Fundamental patterns of knowing in nursing. *Advances in Nursing Science*, Vol. 1, pp13-23.

Castledine, G. (1994) What is clinical supervision? *British Journal of Nursing*, Vol. 3, No. 21, p1135.

Catmur, S. (1995) Clinical supervision in mental health nursing, *Mental Health Nursing*, Vol. 15, No. 1, pp24-25.

Charmaz, K., Mitchell, R.G. (1997) The myth of silent authorship: Self, substance and style in ethnographic writing, in Hertz, R. (ed), *Reflexivity and Voice*, Sage, Thousand Oaks, CA.

Chenitz, W.C., Swanson, J.M. (1986) The Informed Interview, in *From Practice to Grounded Theory*. pp3-15, Addison and Wesley, Wokingham, Berkshire.

Chinn, P.L., Watson, J. (eds) (1994) *Art and Aesthetics in Nursing*, National League for

289

Nursing Press, New York.

Christman, J., Hirshman, J., Holtz, A., Perry, H., Spelkoman, R., Williams, M. (1995) Reflections from the field. Doing Eve's work: Women principals write about their practice, *Anthropology and Education Quarterly*, Vol. 26(2), pp213-227.

Clark, J.A. (1995) Tertiary students' perceptions of their learning environments: A new procedure and some outcomes, *Higher Education Research and Development*, Vol. 14, pp1-12.

Clifford, V.A. (1999) The development of autonomous learners in a university setting, *Higher Education Research and Development*, Vol. 18, No. 1, pp115-128.

Colaizzi, P. (1978) Psychological research as the phenomenologist views it, in Valle, R., King, M. (eds), *Existential Phenomenological Alternatives for Psychology*, Oxford University Press, pp48-71.

Conway, M. (1993) Socialization and roles in nursing, in Werley, M., Fitzpatrick, J. (eds), *Annual Review of Nursing Research*, Springer, New York, pp183-208.

Copp, G. (1997) Patients' and nurses' construction of death and dying in a hospice setting, *Journal of Cancer Nursing*, Vol. 1, No. 1, pp2-13.

Crain, W. (1992) *Theories of Development. Concepts and Applications*, 3rd Edition, Prentice Hall International Inc., New Jersey, pp320-330.

Crotty, M. (1996) *Phenomenology and Nursing Research*, Churchill Livingstone, Australia.

Cumbie, S.A., Rutherford, S.R. (1994) Weaving aesthetics into practice: The use of aesthetic techniques in group psychotherapy with clients remembering repressed traumatic memories, in Chinn, P.L., Watson, J. (1994) (eds), *Art and Aesthetics in Nursing*, National League Co., Nursing Press, New York.

Cushing, A. (1994) Historical and epistemological perspectives on research and nursing, *Journal of Advanced Nursing*, Vol. 20, pp406-411.

Damasio, A. (1994) *Descartes' Error*, New York, Putnam.

Davidson, D. (1986) "A nice derangement of epitaphs.", in Grundy, R., Warner, R., (eds) *Philosophical Grounds of Rationality*, Clarendon Press, Oxford.

Davis, A.J. (1991) The sources of a practice code of ethics for nurses, *Journal of Advanced Nursing*, Nov, Vol. 16, No. 11, pp1358-1362.

Davis, B. (1983) Model students. How students and pupils learn to become nurses, *Nursing Mirror*, Nov 23rd, Vol. 157, No. 21, pp40-41.

Davis, F. (1975) Professional socialization as a subjective experience of the process of doctrinal conversion among student nurses, in Cox, C., Mead, A. (1975) *Sociology of Medical Practice*, Collier Macmillan, London, pp116-131.

Davis-Martin, S. (1990) Research on the difference between baccalaureate and associate degree nurses, *Review of Nursing Research*, Clayton, D., Baj, D. (eds), National League for Nursing, New York.

Davis, B., Sumara, D.J. (1997) Cognition, complexity and teacher education, *Harvard Educational Review*, Vol. 67, pp105-125.

Day, R.A., Field, P.A., Campbell, I.E., Reutter, L. (1995) Students evolving beliefs about nursing from entry to graduation in a four year baccalaureate programme, *Nurse Education Today*, Vol. 15, pp357-364.

Deertz, S. (1978) Conceptualizing human understanding. Gadamers hermeneutics and American communication studies, *Communication Quarterly*, Vol. 26, pp12-23.

Denzin, N.K. (1989) Interpretive Biography, *Qualitative Research Methods*, Vol. 17, Sage Publications, London.

Denzin, N.K., Lincoln, Y. (eds) (1994) *Handbook of Qualitative Research*, Sage Publications, London.

Diekelmann, N. (1990) Notes from Applied Nursing Institute for Interpretive Research Studies. Unpublished raw data, cited in Wilson, H.S., Hutchinson, S.A. (1991) *Qualitative Health Research*, Vol. 1, No. 2, May, pp263-276.

Dilthey, W. (1976) *Dilthey: Selected Writings*, Rickman, H.P. (ed), Cambridge University Press.

Dilworth, D. (1989) *Philosophy in World Perspective. A Comparative Hermeneutic of the Major Theories*, Yale University Press, Newhaven and London.

Donaldson, M. (1992) *Human Minds: An Exploration*, Harmondsworth, Allen Lane.

Dreyfus, H. L. (1987) *Husserl, Heidegger and Modern Existentialism. The Great Philosophers: An Introduction to Western Psychology*, BBC, pp252-274.

Dreyfus, H.L. (1991) *Being in the World. A Commentary on Heidegger's Being and Time*, Division One, The Mit Press, Cambridge, Massachusetts, London, England.

Dreyfus, H.L., Hall, H. (1993) *Heidegger: A Critical Reader*, Blackwell, Oxford, UK.

Eisner, E., Peshkin, R. (1990) *Qualitative Inquiry in Education. The Continuing Debate*, Teachers College Press.

Ellis, C., Flaherty, M. (1992) *Investigating Subjectivity. Research on Lived Experience*, A Sage Focus Edition, Sage Publications, London.

Ellis, R.D., Newton, N. (1998) Three paradoxes of phenomenal consciousness: Bridging the explanatory gap. *Journal of Consciousness Studies*, Vol. 5, No. 4, pp419-442.

Elliston, F., McCormick, M. (eds) (1977) *Husserl; Expositions and Approaches*, University of Notre Dame Press, London.

Evans, P. (1997) *Talking about Nursery Education: Perceptions in Context*, Unpublished PhD thesis, Bristol University.

Fairbairn, G. (1993) How nurses can use a story-telling approach, *Nursing Standard*, April 28th, No. 32, pp32-35.

Feldman, D.C. (1976) A contingency theory and socialisation, *Administrative Science Quarterly*, Vol. 21, pp433-445.

Flagler, S, Loper-Pavers, S., Spitzer, A. (1988) Clinical teaching is more than evaluation alone, *Journal of Nursing Education*, Vol. 27, No. 8, pp342-358.

Ford, K., Jones, A. (1987) *Student Supervision*, Basingstoke, Macmillan.

Fransella, F., Bannister, D. (1977) *A Manual for Repertory Grid Technique*, Academic Press, Harcourt Brace Jovanovich Publishers.

French, P. (1992) The quality of nurse education in the 1980s, *Journal of Advanced Nursing*, Vol. 17, pp610-631.

Gadamer, H.G. (1975) *Truth and Method*, translated by Barders, G., Cumming, J. Sheed and Ward, London.

Gadamer, H.G. (1976) *Philosophical Hermeneutics*, translated and edited by Linge, D. University of California Press, London.

Gadamer, H.G. (1977) *Philosophical Hermeneutics*, translated and edited by Linge, D. University of California Press, Berkeley.

Gadamer, H.G. (1994) *Truth and Method*, Second revised edition. translated and revised by Weinsheimer, J., Marshall, D. Continuum Publishers, New York.

Gagnon, J.H. (1992) cited by Ellis C., Flaherty, M. (eds) in *Investigating Subjectivity*, A Sage Focus Edition, London, Chapter 11, pp221-244.

Gastmans, C. (1998) Interpersonal relations in nursing: A philosophical-ethical analysis of the work of Hildegard E. Peplau, *Journal of Advanced Nursing*, Vol. 28, No. 6, pp1312-1319.

Geanellos, R (1998) Hermeneutic philosophy. Part 1: Implications of its use as methodology in interpretive nursing research, *Nursing Inquiry*, Vol. 5, pp154-163.

Gibbs, G. (1981) *Teaching Students to Learn: A Student-Centred Approach*, OU Press,

Milton Keynes.

Giorgi, A. (1985) (ed) *Phenomenology and Psychological Research*, Duquesne University Press, Pittsburgh.

Glackin, M., Glackin, M. (1998) Investigation into experiences of older students undertaking a pre-registration Diploma in Nursing, *Nurse Education Today*, Vol. 18, pp576-582.

Goffman, E. (1968) *Asylums: Essays on the Social Situation of Patients and the Other Inmates*, Penguin, New York.

Goldenberg, D., Iwasiw, C. (1993) Professional socialization of nursing students as an outcome of a senior clinical preceptorship experience, *Nurse Education Today*, Vol. 13, pp3-15.

Gray, M., Smith, L.N. (1999) The professional socialization of diploma of higher education in nursing students (Project 2000): A longitudinal qualitative study. *Journal of Advanced Nursing*, Vol. 29, No. 3, pp639-647.

Grbich, C. (1990) Socialization and social change: A critique of three positions, *British Journal of Sociology*, Vol. 41, No. 4, pp517-530.

Green, A. (1994) Issues in the application of self-assessment for the Diploma of Higher Education Registered Nurse Mental Health course, *Nurse Education Today*, Vol. 14. pp292-298.

Greenwood, J. (1984) Nursing Research: A position paper, *Journal of Advanced Nursing*, Vol. 9, pp77-82.

Guba, E.G. (ed) (1990) *The Paradigm Dialog*, Newbury Park, CA Sage.

Guba, E.G., Lincoln, Y.S. (1989) *Fourth Generation Evaluation*, Sage Publications, Newbury Park, California.

Guignon, C. (ed) (1996) *The Cambridge Companion to Heidegger*, Cambridge University Press.

Habermas, J. (1971) *Knowledge and Human Interests*, translated by Shapiro, J.J. Boston:Beacon, Pt ii.

Habermas, J. (1987) *The Theory of Communicative Action*, Vol. 2, Polity, Cambridge.

Haggman-Laitila, A. (1999) The authenticity and ethics of phenomenological research: How to overcome the researcher's own views, *Nursing Ethics*, Vol. 6, No. 1, pp12-22.

Hammersley, M., Atkinson, P. (1983) *Ethnography: Principles in Practice*, Tavistock, London.

Hammond, M., Collins, R. (1991) *Self Directed Learning: Critical Practice*, Kogan Page, London.

Hanson, E.J. (1994) Issues concerning the familiarity of researchers within the research setting, *Journal of Advanced Nursing*, Vol. 20, No. 5, pp940-942.

Harre, R. (1983) Identity projects, in Breakwell, G.M. (ed) *Threatened Identities*, Wiley, New York.

Hartman, C.R. (1984) Developing a therapeutic relationship, in Beck, C., Rawlings, R., Williams, S. (eds), *Mental Health - Psychiatric Nursing*, St Louis, Mosby.

Hawkins, P., Shohet, R. (1989) *Supervision for the Helping Professions*, Open University Press, Milton Keynes.

Heidegger, M. (1962) *Being and Time*, translated by Macquarrie, J., Robinson, E. Basil Blackwell, Oxford.

Heidegger, M. (1966) *Discourse on Thinking*, Anderson, J.M., Freund, E.H. (trans), Harper and Row, New York.

Heidegger, M. (1982) *The Basic Problems with Phenomenology*, Indiana University Press.

Heidegger, M. (1997) *Being and Time*, translated by Macquarrie, J., Robinson, E. Blackwell, Oxford.

Hekman, S. (1983) From epistemology to ontology. Gadamers hermeneutics, Wittgensteinian Social Science, *Human Science*, Vol. 6, No. 3, pp205-224.

Helling, I. K. (1988) "The life history method: A survey and a discussion with Norman K. Denzin". *Studies in Symbolic Interaction*, Vol. 9, pp211-243.

Hemsley-Brown, J., Foskett, N.H. (1999) Career desirability: young people's perceptions of nursing as a career, *Journal of Advanced Nursing*, Vol. 29(6), pp1342-1350.

Henderson, V. (1960) *Basic Principles of Nursing Care*, International Council of Nurses, Geneva.

Heyman, R., Shaw, M.P., Harding, J. (1983) A personal construct theory approach to the socialization of nursing trainees in two British general hospitals, *Journal of Advanced Nursing*, Vol. 8, pp50-67.

Hinds, P.S. (1990) Further assessment of a method to estimate reliability and validity of qualitative research findings, *Journal of Advanced Nursing*, Vol. 15, pp430-435.

Holden, R.J. (1991) (1) An analysis of caring: Attributions, contributions and resolutions, *Journal of Advanced Nursing*, Vol. 16, pp893-898.

Holden, R.J. (1991) (2) On applying psychoanalytic explanation in phenomenological research, *International Journal of Nursing Studies*, Vol. 28, No. 4, pp387-396.

Holder, G.M., Jones, R.J., Robinson, R.A., Krass, I. (1999) Academic literary skills and progression rates amongst pharmacy students, *Higher Education Research and Development*, Vol. 18, No. 1, pp19-30.

Holland, R. (1970) George Kelly: Constructive innocent and reluctant existentialist, in Bannister, D. (ed), *Perspectives in Personal Construct Theory*, Academic Press, London.

Holloway, E.L. (1995) *Clinical Supervision: A Systems Approach*, Sage, California.

Holloway, I., Penson, J. (1987) Nurse education as social control, *Nurse Education Today*, Oct, Vol. 7, No. 5, pp235-241.

Holmes, C.A. (1996) The politics of phenomenological concepts in nursing, *Journal of Advanced Nursing*, Vol. 24, pp579-587.

Honderich, T. (ed) (1995) *The Oxford Companion to Philosophy*, Oxford University Press.

House, V.G. (1975) Paradoxes and the undergraduate student nurse, *International Journal of Nursing Studies*, Vol. 12, pp81-86.

Hufton, P. (1996) Give respect where it's due, *Nursing Times*, Oct. 30th, Vol. 92, No. 44, pp59-60.

Hughes, C.A. (1985) Supervising clinical practice in psychosocial nursing, *Journal of Psychosocial Nursing*, Vol. 23, pp27-32.

Husserl, E. (1962) Ideas: *General Introduction to Pure Phenomenology*, Collier, New York.

Husserl, E. (1970) *Logical Investigations*, translated by Findley, J.N. New York, Humanities Press, based on revised Halle edition, Vol. 2, pp446.

Husserl, E. (1991) in Dreyfus, H. *Being in the World. A Commentary on Heidegger's Being and Time*, Division One, The MIT Press, Cambridge, Massachusetts and London, England.

Hyland, M., Millard, J., Parker, S. (1988) How hospital ward members treat learner nurses: An investigation of learner's perceptions in a British hospital, *Journal of Advanced Nursing*, Vol. 13, pp472-477.

James, N. (1992) Care = organisation + physical labour + emotional labour, *Sociology of Health and Illness*, Vol. 14, No. 4, pp488-509.

Jarvis, P. (1983) *Adult and Continuing Education*, Croomhelm, London.

Jasper, M. (1994) Issues in phenomenology for researchers of nursing, *Journal of Advanced Nursing*, Vol. 19, pp309-314.

Johns, C. (1995) The value of reflective practice for nursing, *Journal of Clinical Nursing*, Vol. 4, pp23-30.

Johns, C. (1996) Visualizing and realizing caring in practice through guided reflection, *Journal of Advanced Nursing*, Vol. 24, pp1135-1143.

Johnson, D.E. (1980) The Behavioural System Model for Nursing, in *Conceptual Models for Nursing Practice*, Riehl, J.P., Roy, S.C. (eds), 2nd Edition, Appleton Century Crofts, New York.

Jowett, S. (1995) Nurse education in the 1990s - the implementation of the pre-registration diploma course. (Project 2000), *Nurse Education Today*, Vol. 15, pp39-43.

Jowett, S., Walton, I., Payne, S. (1994) *Challenges and Change in Nurse Education - A Study of the implementation of Project 2000*, National Foundation for Educational Research, Slough, England.

Keen, E. (1975) *A Primer in Phenomenological Psychology*, Holt, Rinehart and Winston, New York, Reprinted in 1982 by University Press of America, Lanham.

Kegan, R. (1996) *The Evolving Self*, Harvard University Press, Cambridge, Massachusetts and London, England.

Keighley, T. (1990) Nurse's homes, *Nursing Times*, Nov. 7th, Vol. 86, No. 45, pp40-41.

Kelly, G.A. (1955) *The Psychology of Personal Constructs*, Norton, New York.

Kelly, G.A. (1970) A brief introduction to personal construct theory, in *Perspectives in Personal Construct Theory*, Bannister, D. (ed), Academic Press, London, pp1-29.

Kelly, G.A. (1977) The psychology of the unknown, in *New Perspectives in Personal Construct theory*, Bannister, D. (ed) Academic Press, London, pp1-19.

Kelly, G.A. (1991) *The Psychology of Personal Constructs. Vol. 1 A Theory of Personality*, Routledge, London.

Kenny, C. (1998) Moonlighting: A student's lot. *Nursing Times*, Feb. 18th, Vol. 94, No. 7, pp29-30.

King, I.M. (1971) *Toward a Theory for Nursing*, John Wiley and Sons, New York. p20.

Kitzinger, J. (1994) The methodology of focus group interviews: The importance of interaction between research participants, *Sociology of Health and Illness*, Vol. 16, No. 1, pp103-121.

Knowles, R.T. (1986) *Human Development and Human Possibility*, University Press of America, Lanham, M.D.

Koch, T. (1994) Establishing rigour in qualitative research: The decision trail, *Journal of Advanced Nursing*, Vol. 19, pp976-986.

Koch, T. (1995) Interpretive approaches in nursing research: The influence of Husserl and Heidegger, *Journal of Advanced Nursing*, Vol. 21, pp827-836.

Koch, T. (1996) Implementation of a hermeneutic enquiry in nursing: Philosophy, rigour and representation, *Journal of Advanced Nursing*, Vol. 24, pp174-184.

Koch, T., Harrington, A. (1998) Reconceptualizing rigour: The case for reflexivity, *Journal of Advanced Nursing*, Vol. 28, No. 4, pp882-890.

Kocklemans, J. (1967) *Phenomenology: The Philosophy of Edmund Husserl and its Interpretation*, Doubleday, New York.

Kocklemans, J. (1986) *A Companion to Martin Heidegger's "Being and Time"*, University Press of America, Washington DC.

Kramer, M. (1974) *Reality Shock: Why Nurses Leave Nursing*, CV Mosby, St Louis.

Kruegar, R.A. (1988) *Focus Groups. A Practical Guide for Applied Research*, Sage publications, London.

Kylma, J., Vehvilainen-Julkunen, K. (1997) Hope in nursing research: A meta-analysis of the ontological and epistemological foundations of research on hope, *Journal of Advanced Nursing*, Vol. 25, pp364-337.

Labor, W., Waletzky, Y. (1966) Narrative analysis: Oral versions of personal experience, in Haler, J. (ed), *Essays on the Verbal and Visual Arts*, American Ethnological Society, Annual Spring Meeting, Washington, pp12-44.

Laing, M. (1993) Gossip: Does it play a role in the socialisation of nurses? *Image: Journal of Nursing Scholarship*, Vol. 25, No. 1, Spring, pp37-43.

Lamb, G.S., Huttlinger, K. (1989) Reflexivity in nursing research, *Western Journal of Nursing Research*, Vol. 11, No. 6, pp765-772.

Lankshear, A. (1998) The cost of caring, *Nursing Times*, Feb. 18th, Vol. 94, No. 7, pp22-23.

Lankshear, A.J. (1993) The use of focus groups in a study of attitudes to student assessment, *Journal of Advanced Nursing*, 18, pp1986-1989.

Lauder, W., Cuthbertson, P. (1998) Course related family and financial problems of mature nursing students, *Nurse Education Today*, Vol. 18, pp419-425.

Laurent, C. (1988) On hand to help, *Nursing Times*, Nov 16th, Vol. 84, No. 46, pp28-30.

Lea, A., Watson, R., Deary, I.J. (1998) Caring in nursing : A multi-variate analysis, *Journal of Advanced Nursing*, Vol. 28, pp662-671.

Leininger, M. (ed) (1988) *Caring: An Essential Human Need*, Wayne State University Press, Detroit, Michigan.

Leonard, V.W. (1989) A Heideggerian phenomenologic perspective of the concept of the person, *Advances in Nursing Science*, July, Vol. 11, No. 4, pp40-55.

Lincoln, Y., Guba, E. (1985) *Naturalistic Inquiry*, Sage Publications, Newbury Park.

Lipson, J. (1997) On bracketing, in Morse, J. (ed) *Qualitative Nursing Research: A Contemporary Dialogue*, Sage Publications, Newbury Park, pp23-24.

Lofland, J., Lofland, L.H. (1984) *Analysing Social Settings: A Guide to Qualitative Observation and Analysis*, 2nd edition, Wadsworth, Belmont.

Loftus, L.A. (1998) Student nurses' lived experience of the sudden death of their patients, *Journal of Advanced Nursing*, Vol. 27, pp641-648.

Louis, M.R. (1980) Surprise and sense making: What newcomers experience in entering unfamiliar organizational settings, *Administrative Science Quarterly*, Vol. 25, No. 2, pp226-251.

Luker, K.A. (1984) Reading nursing: the burden of being different, *International Journal of Nursing Studies*, Vol. 21, No. 1, pp1-7.

Lum, J.L.J. (1988) Reference groups and professional socialisation, in Hardy, M.E., Conway, M.E., *Role Theory: Perspectives for Health Professionals*, 2nd edition, Appleton and Lange, Norwalk CT, pp137-156.

Macleod Clark, J., Maben, J., Jones, K. (1996) *Project 2000: Perceptions of the Philosophy and Practice of Nursing*, The Nightingale Institute, Kings College, London, ENB, London.

Macleod, M. (1994) "It's the little things that count": The hidden complexity of everyday clinical nursing practice, *Journal of Clinical Nursing*, Vol. 3, pp361-368.

Maltby, H., Drury, J., Fischer-Rasmussen, V. (1995) The roots of nursing: teaching caring based on Watson, *Nurse Education Today*, Vol. 15, pp44-46.

Manninen, E. (1998) Changes in nursing students' perceptions of nursing as they progress through their education, *Journal of Advanced Nursing*, Vol. 27, pp390-398.

Manusov, V., Rodriguez, J., Scott, (1989) Intentionality behind non-verbal messages: A practitioner's perspective, *Journal of Non-Verbal Behaviour*, Vol. 13, No. 1, pp15-24.

Markus, H., Nurius, P. (1986) Possible selves, *American Psychologist*, Sept, Vol. 41, No. 9, pp954-969.

Maslow, A.H. (1954) *Motivation and Personality*, Harper and Row, New York.

Maslow, A.H. (1968) *Toward a Psychology of Being*, 2nd edition, Van Nostrand Reinhold, New York.

Maslow, A.H. (1970) *Motivation and Personality*, 3rd edition, Harper Collins Publishers, London.

May, K.A. (1991) Interview techniques in qualitative research: Concerns and challenges, in Morse, J.M. (ed), *Qualitative Nursing Research: A Contemporary Dialogue*, CA Sage, Newbury Park, pp188-201.

May, N., Veitch, L., McIntosh, J.B., Alexander, M.F. (1997) *Preparation for Practice. Evaluation of Nurse and Midwife Education in Scotland. 1992 Programmes*, Department of Nursing and Community Health, Glasgow Caledonian University, Glasgow.

May, R. (1969) *Love and Will*, Souvenir Press, London.

McCall, G.J., Simmons, J.E. (1978) *Identities and Intentions*, 2nd edition, Free Press, New York.

McEvoy, C. (1995) *The Report of the Summative Evaluation of Project 2000 in Northern Ireland*, National Board for Nursing Midwifery and Health Visiting for Northern Ireland.

McKay, J., Emmison, M. (1995) Using learner-centred learning (LCL) in undergraduate sociology courses, *ANZ Journal of Sociology*, Vol. 31, No. 3, pp94-103.

McQuarrie, E.F., McIntyre, S.H. (1987) What focus groups can and cannot do. A reply to Seymour, *Journal of Product Innovation Management*, Vol. 4, pp55-60.

Melia, K.M. (1981) *Student Nurses' Accounts of Their Work and Training. A Qualitative analysis*, Unpublished PhD thesis, University of Edinburgh.

Melia, K.M. (1984) Student nurses' construction of occupational socialization, *Sociology of Health and Illness*, Vol. 6, No. 2, pp133-150.

Melia, K.M. (1987) *Learning and Working. The Occupational Socialization of Nurses*, Tavistock Publications.

Mendelson, J. (1979) The Habermas - Gadamer debate, *New German Critique*, Vol. 18, pp44-73.

Mendes de Almeida, (1980) A review of group discussion methodology, *European Research*, Vol. 8, No. 3, pp114-120.

Merleau-Ponty, M. (1948) Sens et non-sens. (Paris Nagel, 1948, p261) *Sense and Nonsense*, translation in Dreyfus, Dreyfus, (1964) Evanston, North Western University Press, p148.

Merleau-Ponty, M. (1962) *The Phenomenology of Perception*, Routledge and Kegan-Paul, London.

Merleau-Ponty, M. (1964) *The Primacy of Perception*, North-Western University Press, Evanston, Il., p49.

Miles, M.B., Huberman, A.M. (1994) *Qualitative Data Analysis: A Sourcebook of New Methods*, Beverley Hills, CA Sage Publications.

Miller, M.P. (1981) *A Phenomenological Investigation of the Creative Process of Women Poets*, Unpublished doctoral dissertation, California School of Professional Psychology, Berkeley, CA.

Mitchell, T. (1999) Present tense commentary: A qualitative research technique, *Nurse*

Education Today, Feb., Vol. 19, No. 2, pp151-158.

Moore, J.R., Gilbert, D.A. (1995) Elderly residents: Perceptions of nurses' comforting touch, *Journal of Gerontological Nursing*, Vol. 21, No. 1, pp6-13.

Morgan, D.L. (1988) Focus groups as qualitative research, A Sage University Paper, *Qualitative Research Methods*, Series 16.

Morrison, P. (1990) An example of the use of repertory grid technique in assessing nurse self perceptions of caring, *Nurse Education Today*, Vol. 10, pp253-259.

Morrison, P. (1991) The caring attitude in nursing practice: A repertory grid study of trained nurses' perceptions, *Nurse Education Today*, Vol. 11, pp3-12.

Morrow, R.A. (1994) *Critical Theory and Methodology*, Vol. 3, Sage Publications, London.

Mortimer, J.T., Simmons, R.G. (1978) Adult socialization, *Annual Review of Sociology*, Vol. 4, pp421-454.

Moustakas, C. (1994) *Phenomenological Research Methods*, Sage Publications Inc., London.

Mulhall, S. (1990) *On Being in the World: Wittgenstein and Heidegger on Seeing Aspects*, Routledge and Kegan Paul, London.

Munhall, P. (1994) *Revisioning Phenomenology: Nursing and Health Science Research*, National League for Nursing Press, New York.

Natanson, M. (1974) *Phenomenology, Role and Reason. Essays on the Coherence and Deformation of Social Reality*, Charles C. Thomas, Springfield, Illinois.

Natsoulas,T. (1992) Intentionality, consciousness and subjectivity, *Journal of Mind and Behaviour*, Vol.13(3), pp281-308.

Neimeyer, G., Neimeyer, R. (1985) Relational trajectories: a personal construct contribution, *Journal of Social and Personal Relationships*, Vol. 2, pp325-349.

Nelms, T.P. (1996) Living a caring presence in nursing: A Heideggerian hermeneutic analysis, *Journal of Advanced Nursing*, Vol. 24, pp368-374.

Nolan, P., Brown, B., Crawford, P. (1998) Fruits without labour: The implications of Friedrich Nietzshe's ideas for the caring professions, *Journal of Advanced Nursing*, Vol. 28, No. 2, pp251-259.

Nyamathi, A., Schuler, P. (1990) Focus group interviews: A research technique for informed nursing practice, *Journal of Advanced Nursing*, Vol. 15, pp1281-1288.

Oleson, V., Whitaker, E. (1968) *The Silent Dialogue: A Study of the Social Psychology of Professional Socialization*, Jossey Bass, San Francisco.

Olsson, H.M., Gullberg, M.T. (1987) Nursing education and professional role acquisition - theoretical perspectives, *Nurse Education Today*, Vol. 7, No. 4, pp171-176.

Omery, A. (1983) Phenomenology: a method for nursing research, *Advances in Nursing Science*, Vol. 5, No. 2, pp47-63.

O'Neill, E., Morrison, H., McEwen, A. (1993) *Professional Socialization and Nurse Education: An Evaluation*, Executive Summary, The Queens University of Belfast.

Orem, D.E. (1980) *Nursing: Concepts of Practice*, McGraw-Hill Book Co., New York.

Packer, M.J., Addison, R.B. (eds) (1989) *Entering the Circle. Hermeneutic Investigation in Psychology*, State University of New York Press.

Packwood, A., Sikes, P. (1996) Adopting a post-modernist approach to research, *International Journal of Qualitative Studies in Education*, Vol. 9, No. 3, pp335-345.

Parker, T.J., Carlisle, C. (1996) Project 2000 students' perceptions of their training, *Journal of Advanced Nursing*, Vol. 24, pp771-778.

Parse, R.R. (1981) *Man-Living-Health: A Theory of Nursing*, John Wiley and Sons, New

York.

Parse, R.R. (1990) Parse's research methodology with an illustration of the lived experience of hope, *Nursing Science Quarterly*, Vol. 3, No. 1, pp9-17.

Parse, R.R. (1992) Human becoming: Parse's theory of nursing, *Nursing Science Quarterly*, Vol. 5, pp35-42.

Parse, R.R. (1993) The experience of laughter: A phenomenological study, *Nursing Science Quarterly*, Vol. 6, No. 1, pp39-43.

Paterson, B.L., Crawford, M., Saydak, M., Venkatesh, P., Tschikota, W.S., Aronowitz, T. (1995) How male nursing students learn to care, *Journal of Advanced Nursing*, Vol. 22, pp600-609.

Peplau, H.E. (1952) *Interpersonal Relations in Nursing*, Putnam, New York.

Peplau, H.E. (1988) The art and science of nursing. Similarities, differences and relations, *Nursing Science quarterly*, Vol. 1, No. 1, pp8-15.

Peplau, H.E. (1994) Quality of life. An interpersonal perspective, *Nursing Science Quarterly*, Vol. 7, No. 1, pp10-15.

Peplau, H.E. (1996) Transforming practice knowledge into nursing knowledge. A revisionist analysis of Peplau, *Image: Journal of Nursing Scholarship*, Vol. 29, No. 1, pp29-33.

Philpin, S. (1999) The impact of Project 2000 educational reforms on the occupational socialisation of nurses: An exploratory study, *Journal of Advanced Nursing*, Vol. 29, No. 6, pp1326-1331.

Pickles, J. (1985) *Phenomenology, Science and Geography: Spatiality and the Human Sciences*, Cambridge University Press, Cambridge.

Pierson, W. (1998) Reflection and nursing education, *Journal of Advanced Nursing*, Vol. 27, pp165-170.

Pilhammar-Anderson, E. (1993) The perspective of student nurses and their perceptions of professional nursing during the nurse training programme, *Journal of Advanced Nursing*, Vol. 18, pp808-815.

Plant, L. (1993) Unsafe as houses? *Nursing Times*, Nov. 17th, Vol. 89, No. 46, pp36-37.

Pollock, L.C. (1986) An introduction to the use of repertory grid technique as a research method and clinical tool for psychiatric nurses, *Journal of Advanced Nursing*, Vol. 11, pp439-445.

Porter, L.W., Lawler, E.E., Hackman, R.J. (1975) *Behaviour Organisations*, McGraw-Hill, New York.

Price, B. (1986) A clash of characters, *Nursing Times*, Jan. 29th, pp40-42.

Pritchard, J (ed) (1995) *Good Practice and Supervision*, Jessica Kingsley Publishers, pp193-201.

Ramos, M.C. (1989) Some ethical implications of qualitative research, *Research in Nursing and Health*, Vol. 12, pp57-63.

Ramprogus, V. (1995) *The Deconstruction of Nursing*, Avebury, Aldershot.

Ramsay, S., Barker, M., Jones, E. (1999) Academic adjustment and learning processes: a comparison of international and local students in first year university, *Higher Education Research and Development*, Vol. 18, No. 1, pp129-144.

Ravey, D. (1992) *Mentors, Preceptors and Supervisors: Their Place in Nursing, Midwifery and Health Visiting Education*, Welsh National Board, Cardiff.

Rawlinson, J. (1995) Some reflections on the use of repertory grid technique in studies of nurses and social workers, *Journal of Advanced Nursing*, Vol. 21, pp334-339.

Ray, M. (1990) Phenomenological method for nursing research, in Chaska, N. (ed), *The Nursing Profession: Turning Points*, McGraw - Hill, New York, pp173-178.

Reason, P., Rowan, J (eds) (1981) *Human Inquiry: A Sourcebook of New Paradigm*

Research, John Wiley, Chichester, UK.

Reed, J., Roskell, V. (1997) Focus Groups: Issues of analysis and interpretation, *Journal of Advanced Nursing*, 26, pp765-771.

Reinharz, S. (1983) Experiential analysis: a contribution to feminist research, in Baule, G., Klein, B. (eds), *Theories of Womens Studies*, Routledge and Kegan Paul, London.

Richardson, L. (1990) *Writing Strategies - Reaching Diverse Audiences*, Sage Publications Inc, London.

Richardson, L. (1992) The consequences of poetic representation. Writing the other, rewriting the self, in, Ellis, C., Flaherty, M. *Investigating Subjectivity*, A Sage focus Edition, Chapter 6, pp125-137.

Richardson, L. (1994) Nine-poems: marriage and the family, *Journal of Contemporary Ethnography*, Vol. 23, No. 1, pp3-13.

Roach, S. (1992) *The Human Act of Caring*, Revised edition, Canadian Hospital Association Press, Ottawa.

Roberts, S., McGinty, S. (1995) Reflections from the field. Awareness of presence: Developing the researcher self, *Anthropology and Education Quarterly*, Vol. 26, No. 1, pp112-122.

Robinson, J.E. (1991) *Experiences of a Project 2000 Demonstration District*, Ipswich, SGY CNM.

Rogers, C. (1942) *Counselling and Psychotherapy. New Concepts in Practice*, Houghton Mifflin, Boston.

Rolfe, G. (1990) The role of clinical supervision in the education of student psychiatric nurses: A theoretical approach, *Nurse Education Today*, Vol. 10, pp193-197.

Roper, N., Logan, W.W., Tierney, A.J. (1985) *The Elements of Nursing*, Churchill Livingstone, Edinburgh.

Rosaldo, M. (1984) "Toward an anthropology of self feeling", in Schweder, R.A., Levine, R.A. (eds), *Culture Theory: Essays on Mood, Self and Emotion*, Cambridge, Cambridge University Press.

Rose, J.F. (1990) Psychologic health of women: a phenomenologic study of women's inner strength, *Advances in Nursing Science*, January, Vol. 12, No. 2, pp56-70.

Rose, P., Beeby, J., Parker, D. (1995) Academic rigour in the lived experience of researchers using phenomenological methods in nursing, *Journal of Advanced Nursing*, Vol. 21, pp1123-1129.

Routasalo, P., Isola, A. (1996) The right to touch and be touched, *Nursing Ethics*, Vol. 3, No. 2, pp165-176.

Sandelowski, M. (1986) The problem with rigour in qualitative research, *Advances in Nursing Science*, Vol. 8, p27.

Sandelowski, M. (1991) Telling stories: Narrative approaches in qualitative research, *Image: Journal of Nursing Scholarship*, Vol. 23, No. 3, pp161-165.

Sartre, J.P. (1969) *Being and Nothingness*, University Paperback, London.

Sartre, J.P. (1978) *Being and Nothingness*, Simon and Schuster, New York.

Sartre, J.P. (1996) *Being and Nothingness*. Routledge, London.

Schlenker, B.R. (1980) *Impression Management: The Self Concept, Social Identity and Interpersonal Relations*, Brooks/Cole:Monterey CA.

Schoenhofer, S.O. (1989) Affectional touch in critical nursing: A descriptive study, *Heart and Lung*, Vol. 18. pp146-154.

Scholes, J., Freeman, M. (1994) The reflective dialogue and repertory grid: a research approach to identify the unique contribution of nursing, midwifery or health visiting to the therapeutic milieu, *Journal of Advanced Nursing*, Vol. 20, pp885-893.

Schon, D.A. (1983) *The Reflective Practitioner: How Professionals Think in Action*, New York Basic Books.

Schon, D.A. (1987) *Educating the Reflective Practitioner*, Jossey-Bass Publishers, London.

Schutz, A. (1994) Exploring the benefits of a subjective approach in qualitative nursing research, *Journal of Advanced Nursing*, Vol. 20, pp412-417.

Scully, R. (1980) Stress in the nurse, cited by Severinsson, E.I., Borgenhammar, E.V. (1997) Expert views on clinical supervision. A study based on interviews, *Journal of Nursing Management*, Vol. 5, pp175-183.

Seccombe, I., Jackson, C., Patch, A. (1995) *Nursing: The Next Generation*, Institute for Employment Studies, Report 344.

Seed, A. (1991) *Becoming a Registered Nurse - The Students Perspective*, Unpublished PhD. Thesis, Leeds polytechnic.

Severinsson, E. (1996) Nurse supervisors views of their supervisory styles in clinical supervision. A hermeneutical approach, *Journal of Nursing Management*, Vol. 4, pp191-199.

Seymour, J.E., Ingleton, C. (1999) Ethical issues in qualitative research at the end of life, *International Journal of Palliative Nursing*, Vol. 5, No. 2, pp65-73.

Shead, H. (1991) Role conflict in student nurses: Toward a positive approach for the 1990s, *Journal of Advanced Nursing*, Vol. 16, pp736-740.

Silverman, H.J (ed) (1991) *Answers to Critical Theory. Gadamer and Hermeneutics*, Routledge, New York and London, p161.

Simpson, I.H. (1979) *From Student to Nurse: A Longitudinal Study of Socialisation*, Cambridge University Press, New York.

Smith, K.V. (1996) Ethical decision-making in nursing: Implications for continuing education, *The Journal of Continuing Education in Nursing*, Vol. 27, No. 1, pp42-45.

Smithers, A., Griffin, A. (1986) Mature students at university: Entry experience and outcomes, *Studies in Higher Education*, Vol. 11, No. 3, pp257-268.

Sourial, S. (1997) An analysis of caring, *Journal of Advanced Nursing*, Vol. 26, pp1189-1192.

Spiegelberg, H. (1960) *The Phenomenological Movement*, Martinus Nijhoff, The Hague.

Spiegelberg, H. (1969) *The Phenomenological Movement. A Historical Introduction*, 2nd edition, Vol. Two, Martinus Nijhoff, The Hague.

Spiegelberg, H. (1982) *The Phenomenological Movement. A Historical Introduction*, 3rd edition, Martinus Nijhoff, Boston.

Spouse, J. (1996) The effective mentor: A model for student centred learning in clinical practice, *Nursing Times Research*, Vol. 1, No. 2, pp120-133.

Stacey, J. (1988) Can there be a feminist ethnography? *Women's Studies International Forum*, Vol. 11, No. 1, pp21-27.

Stark, S., Redding, M. (1993) A profile of part time students, *Senior Nurse*, Vol. 13, No. 4, pp48-52.

Stern, L. (1985) Hermeneutics and intellectual history, *Journal of the History of Ideas*, Vol. 46, April/June, pp287-296.

Stevens, R. (ed) (1996) *Understanding Self*, The Open University, Sage Publications, London.

Stewart, J. (1995) Merleau-Ponty's criticisms of Sartre's theory of freedom, *Philosophy Today*, Fall, pp311-324.

Stiles, W.B. (1993) Quality control, in qualitative research, *Clinical Psychology Review*, Vol. 13, pp593-618.

Street, A.F. (1992) *Inside Nursing. A Critical Ethnography of Clinical Nursing Practice*, State University of New York Press, Albany, New York.

Stringer, O., Bannister, D. (1979) Introduction, in Stringer, P., Bannister, D. (eds), *Constructs of Sociality and Individuality*, Academic, London.

Swanson, D.L., Delia, J.G. (1976) *The Nature of Human Communication*, Science Research Associates, Chicago.

Tattam, A. (1990) Homes fit for nurses? *Nursing Times*, Oct. 3rd, Vol. 86, No. 40, pp28-31.

Taylor, B. (1993) Phenomenological: One way to understand nursing practice, *International Journal of Nursing Studies*, Vol. 30, No. 2, pp171-179.

Taylor, B.J. (1994) *Being Human: Ordinariness in Nursing*, Churchill Livingstone, Melbourne.

Thomas, L.F., Harri-Augstein, E.S. (1985) *Self Organised Learning: Foundations of a Conversational Science for Psychology*, Routledge and Kegan Paul, London.

Thompson, J. 1994. *Hermeneutics and its Shadow: Contradictions of Tradition and Community in Nursing*, Unpublished seminar paper, school of nursing, University of Southern Maine, Portland, Maine.

Tilley, S., Chambers, M. (1996) Research in brief. Problems of the researching person: doing insider research with your peer group, *Journal of Psychiatric and Mental Health Nursing*, Vol. 3, pp267-268.

Twinn, S. (1992) Issues in the supervision of health visiting practice: An agenda for debate, in Butterworth, T., Faugier, J. (eds) *Clinical Supervision and Mentorship in Nursing*, Chapman and Hall, London, pp132-143.

United Kingdom Central Council (1986) *Project 2000: A New Preparation for Practice*, UKCC, London.

United Kingdom Central Council (1992) *Code of Professional Conduct*, 3rd edition, UKCC, London.

United Kingdom Central Council (1999) *Fitness for Practice. The UKCC Commission for Nursing and Midwifery Education*, The Peach Report, UKCC, London.

Usher, K., Arthur, D. (1998) Process consent: A model for enhancing informed consent in mental health nursing, *Journal of Advanced Nursing*, Vol. 27, pp692-697.

Usher, K., Holmes, C. (1997) Ethical aspects of phenomenological research with mentally ill people, *Nursing Ethics*, Vol. 4, No. 1, pp49-56.

Valle, R.S., Halling, S. (eds) (1989) *Existential Phenomenological Perspectives in Psychology*, Plenum Press, New York and London.

Van Kaam, A. (1966) *Existential Foundations of Psychology*, Duquesne Studies Psychological Series 3, Duquesne University Press, Pittsburgh.

Van Maanen, J. (1976) Breaking in, in Belcher and Atchison, *Socialisation to Work*, pp67-130.

Van Maanen, J. (1988) *Tales of the Field. On Writing Ethnography*, The University of Chicago Press, Chicago and London.

Van Manen, M. (1990) *Researching Lived Experience*, T. Althouse, London and Ontario.

Van Manen, M. (1991) Reflexivity and the pedagogical moment: The normativity of pedagogical thinking and acting, *Journal of Curriculum Studies*, Vol. 23, No. 6, pp507-536.

Van Manen, M. (1996) *From Meaning to Method*, Paper presented at the Qualitative Health Research conference, Oct 30th, Bournemouth, UK.

Vezeau, T.M. (1992) *Narrative Inquiry in Nursing: Issues and Original Works*, University microfilms international.

Vezeau, T.M. (1993) Storytelling: a practitioners tool, *Mother and Child Nursing*, Vol.

18, July/Aug, pp193-196.

Visker, R. (1991) From Foucault to Heidegger: A one-way ticket? *Research in Phenomenology*, Vol. 21, pp116-140.

Walsh, K. (1996) Philosophical hermeneutics and the project of Hans Georg Gadamer. Implications for nurse researchers, *Nursing Inquiry*, Vol. 3, pp231-237.

Walters, A.J. (1995) The phenomenological movement: Implications for nursing research, *Journal of Advanced Nursing*, Vol. 22, pp791-799.

Warnke, G. (1987) *Gadamer: Hermeneutics, Tradition and Reason*, Polity Press, Cambridge.

Watson, J. (1979) *Nursing: The Philosophy and Science of Caring*, Little, Brown and Co, Boston.

Watson, J. (1985) *Human Science and Human Care: A Theory of Nursing*, Appleton-Century-Crofts, Norwalk, CT.

Watson, J. (1988) *Nursing: Human Science and Human Care. A Theory of Nursing*, National League for Nursing, New York.

Watson, R., Deary, I.J., Lea, A. (1999) A longitudinal study into the perceptions of caring and nursing among nurses, *Journal of Advanced Nursing*, Vol. 29, No. 5, pp1228-1237.

Watson, R., Lea, A. (1997) The caring dimensions inventory (CDI): Content validity, reliability and scaling, *Journal of Advanced Nursing*, Vol. 25, pp87-94.

Webb, C. (1992) The use of the first person in academic writing: objectivity, language and gatekeeping, *Journal of Advanced Nursing*, Vol. 17, pp747-752.

Weedon, C. (1987) *Feminist Practice and Post Structuralist Theory*, Basil Blackwell, New York.

Weiss, S. (1986) Psychophysiologic effects of caregiver touch on incidence of cardiac dysrhythmia, *Heart and Lung*, Vol. 15, pp495-505.

Wetherick, N. (1970) Can there be a non-phenomenological psychology? *Journal of the British Society for Phenomenology*, Vol. 1, pp72-80.

Wheeler, S., Birtle, J. (1993) *A Handbook of Personal Students*, Open University Press, Milton Keynes, pp83-102.

While, A. (1991) The problem of clinical evaluation: A review, *Nurse Education Today*, Vol. 11, pp448-453.

White, A. (1996) A theoretical framework created from a repertory grid analysis of graduate nurse's in relation to the feelings they experience in clinical practice, *Journal of Advanced Nursing*, Vol. 24, pp144-150.

White, E., Riley, E., Davies, S., Twinn, S. (1993) *A Detailed Study of the Relationships Between Teaching, Support, Supervision and Role Modelling for Students in Clinical Areas Within the Context of Project 2000*, Kings College London and University of Manchester, ENB.

Whitmarsh, J. (1993) Opening the door to opportunity, *Nursing Times*, May 19th, Vol. 89, No. 20, pp36-37.

Wilde, V. (1992) Controversial hypotheses on the relationship between researcher and informant in qualitative research, *Journal of Advanced Nursing*, Vol. 17, pp234-242.

Wilkinson, D. (1982) The effects of brief psychiatric training on the attitudes of general nursing students of psychiatric patients, *Journal of Advanced Nursing*, Vol. 7, pp239-253.

Wilson-Barnett, J., Butterworth, T., White, E., Twinn, S., Davies, S., Riley, L. (1995) Clinical support and the Project 2000 nursing student: Factors influencing this process, *Journal of Advanced Nursing*, 21, pp1152-1158.

Wilson, H.S., Hutchinson, S.A. (1991) Pearls, pith and provocations. Triangulation of qualitative methods: Heideggerian hermeneutics and grounded theory, *Qualitative Health Research*, Vol. 1, No. 2, May, pp263-276.

Wilson, A., Startup, R. (1991) Nurse socialisation: Issues and problems, *Journal of Advanced Nursing*, Dec, Vol. 16, No. 12, pp1478-1486.

Witkin, R. (1994) Running a commentary on imaginatively relived events: A technique for obtaining qualitatively rich discourse, *British Journal of Sociology*, No. 45, Issue No. 2, June, pp265-285.

Wolfer, J. (1993) Aspects of "reality" and ways of knowing in nursing: In search of an integrating paradigm, *Image: Journal of Nursing Scholarship*, Vol. 25, pp141-146.

Wong, F., Kember, D., Chung, L., Yan, L. (1995) Assessing the level of student reflection from reflective journals, *Journal of Advanced Nursing*, Vol. 22, pp48-57.

Wong, J., Wong, S. (1987) Towards effective clinical teaching in nursing, *Journal of Advanced Nursing*, Vol. 12, pp505-513.

Wood, V. (1982) Evaluation of student nurse clinical performance: A continuing problem, *International Nursing Review*, Vol. 29, No. 1, pp11-18.

Woods, P. (1999) *Successful Writing for Qualitative Researchers*, Routledge, London and New York.

Wrigley, K.M. (1995) Constructed selves, constructed lives: A cultural constructivist perspective of mental health nursing practice, *Journal of Psychiatric and Mental Health Nursing*, Vol. 2, pp97-103.

Wyatt J.F. (1978) Sociological perspectives on socialisation into a profession: A study of student nurses and their definition of learning, *British Journal of Educational Studies*, Vol. XXVl, No. 3, October, pp263-276.

Younger, J. (1990) Literary works as a mode of knowing, *Image: Journal of Nursing Scholarship*, Vol. 22, Spring, pp39-43.

Bibliography

Bibliography

Addison, R.B. (1984) *Surviving the Residency: A Grounded Interpretive Investigation*, University Microfilms International (1985), PhD Thesis, University of California, Berkeley.

Addison, R.B. (1989) Grounded interpretive research: An investigation of physician socialization, in Packer and Addison (eds), *Entering the Circle*, State University of New York Press, Chapter 1, pp39-58.

Alten, D.G. (1995) Heremeutics: Philosophical traditions and nursing practice research, *Nursing Science Quarterly*, Vol. 8, No 4, Winter, pp174-182.

Alten, M.N., Jensen, L. (1990) Hermeneutic enquiry: Meaning and scope, *Western Journal of Nursing Research*, Vol. 12, pp241-253.

Anderson, J.M. (1991) Reflexivity in Fieldwork: Toward a feminist epistemology, *Image: Journal of Nursing Scholarship*, Vol. 23, Summer, pp115-118.

Argyle, M. (1973) *Social Interaction*, Methuen, London.

Armstrong, E.G. (1976) On phenomenology and sociological theory, *British Journal of Sociology*, Vol. 27, No. 2, June, pp251-253.

Arthur, D. (1992) Measuring the professional self-concept of nurses: A critical review, *Journal of Advanced Nursing*, Vol. 17, No. 6, June, pp712-719.

Ashworth, P.D. (1979) *Social Interaction and Consciousness*, Wiley, Chichester.

Attig, T. (1992) Person centred death education, *Death Studies*, Vol. 16, pp357-370.

Avis, M. (1995) Valid Arguments? A consideration of the concept of validity in establishing the credibility of research findings, *Journal of Advanced Nursing*, Vol. 22, pp1203-1209.

Babbie, E. (1979) *The Practice of Social Research*, 3rd edition, Wadsworth, Belmot, California.

Baillie, L. (1993) Factors affecting student nurses' learning in community placements: A phenomenological study, *Journal of Advanced Nursing*, Vol. 18, pp1043-1053.

Baker, C., Wvest, J., Noeragerstern, P. (1992) Method slurring: The grounded theory, phenomenology example, *Journal of Advanced Nursing*, Vol. 17, pp1355-1360.

Bandura cited in Crain, W. (1992) *Theories of Development: Concepts and Applications. Bandura's Social Learning Theory*, Prentice Hall International Inc., pp175-192.

Bartlett, W.E. (1983) Major contributions - Part One: The framework. A multidimensional framework for the analysis of supervision of counselling, *The Counselling Psychologist*, Vol. 11, No. 1, pp9-17.

Bassett, C. (1993) Socialization of student nurses into the qualified nurses role. *British Journal of Nursing*, Vol. 2, No. 3, pp179-182.

Beck, C.T. (1992) The lived experience of post partem depression: A phenomenological study, *Nursing Research*, Vol. 14, No. 3, pp166-170.

Beck, C.T. (1993) Qualitative research: The evaluation of its credibility, fittingness and auditability, *Western Journal of Nursing Research*, Vol. 15, No. 2, pp283-266.

Becker, H.S. (1968) The self and adult socialization, in Norbeck, E., Price-Williams, D., McCord, W.M. (eds), *The Study of Personality*, Holt, Rinehart and Winston, New

York.

Begat, I.B.E., Severinsson, E.I., Berggren, I.B. (1997) Implementation of clinical supervision in a medical department: Nurses views of the effects, *Journal of Clinical Nursing*, Vol. 6, pp389-394.

Berger, P.L., Luckman, T. (1979) *The Social Construction of Reality*, Penguin Books, Middlesex.

Betz, C. (1985) Students in transition: Imitators or role models, *Journal of Nursing Education*, Vol. 24, No. 7, pp301-303.

Blumer, H. (1965-6) Sociological Implications of the thought of George Herbert Mead (Symbolic Interactionism), *American Journal of Sociology*, Vol. 71, pp535-44.

Bottoroff, J.L., Gogag, M., Engelberg-Lotzkar, M. (1995) Comforting: Exploring the work of cancer nurses, *Journal of Advanced Nursing*, Vol. 22, pp1077-1084.

Boud, D.J. (1992) The use of self-assessment schedules in negotiated learning, *Studies in Higher Education*, Vol. 17, No. 2, p185-200.

Bourdieu, P. (1991) *The Political Ontology of Martin Heidegger*, Stanford University Press, Standford, California.

Bowles, N. (1995) Story-telling: A search for meaning within nursing practice, *Nurse Education Today*, Vol. 15, pp365-369.

Bracken, E., Davis, J. (1989) The implications of mentorship in nursing career development, *Senior Nurse*, Vol. 9, No. 5, May, pp15-16.

Braithwaite, D.N., Elzubeir, M., Stark, S. (1994) Project 2000 student wastage: A case study, *Nurse Education Today*, Vol. 14, pp15-21.

Brand, G. (1967) Intentionality, reduction and intentional analysis in Husserls later manuscripts, in Kockelmans, J.J. (ed), *Phenomenology*, Garden City, Doubleday, N.Y., pp197-217.

Brandt, L.W. (1970) Phenomenology, psychoanalysis and behaviourism, (E = S), *Journal of Phenomenological Psychology*, Vol. 1, pp7-18.

Brink, P. (1987) On reliability and validity in qualitative research, *Western Journal of Nursing Research*, Vol. 2, pp157-159.

Brock, S.C., Kleiber, D.A. (1994) Narrative in Medicine: The stories of elite college athletes' career ending injuries, *Qualitative Health Research*, Vol. 4, No. 4, Nov., pp411-430.

Brodbeck, M. (1968) *Readings in the Philosophy of the Social Sciences*, University of Minnesota, The Macmillan Co., London.

Bunting, S. (1993) *Rosemarie Parse: Theory of Health and Becoming*, Sage Publications, London.

Burgess, R.G. (1984) *In the Field*, Allen and Unwin, London.

Butterworth, T., Bishop, V., Carson, J. (1996) First steps towards evaluating clinical supervision in nursing and health visiting, 1. Theory, policy and practice development: A review, *Journal of Clinical Nursing*, Vol. 5, pp127-132.

Cain, W. (1992) *Theories of Development. Concepts and Applications*, Prentice Hall, International Inc.

Campbell, J.C., Bunting, S. (1991) Voices and Paradigms: Perspectives on critical and feminist theory in nursing, *Advances in Nursing Science*, Vol. 13, No. 3, pp1-15.

Carspeckon, P.F., Cordeiro, P.A. (1995) Being, Doing and Becoming: Textural interpretations of social identity and a case study, in *Qualitative Inquiry*, Vol.1, No.1, Sage Publications Inc., pp87-109.

Catalano, J.S. (1985) *A Commentary on Jean-Paul Sartre's 'Being and Nothingness'*, University of Chicago Press.

Chambers, M. (1995) Supportive clinical supervision: A crucible for personal and professional change, *Journal of Psychiatric and Mental Health Nursing*, Vol. 2, pp311-316.

Christmam, L. (1991) Perspectives on Role. Socialization of Nurses, *Nursing Outlook*, Vol. 39(5), Sept-Oct., pp209-212.

Clausen, J.A. (ed) (1968) *Socialization and Society*, Little, Brown and Co., Boston.

Clayton, G.M., Broome, H.E., Ellis, L.A. (1989) Relationship between preceptorship experience and role socialization of graduate nurses, *Journal of Nursing Education*, Vol. 28, No. 2, pp72-75.

Cohen, J.A. (1991) Two portraits of caring: A comparison of the artists, Leininger and Watson, *Journal of Advanced Nursing*, Vol. 16, pp899-909.

Cohen, M. (1987) A historical overview of the phenomenological movement, *Image: Journal of Nursing Scholarship*, Vol. 19, No. 1, pp31-34.

Conway, M. (1993) Socialization and roles in nursing, in Werley, M., Fitzpatrick, J. (eds), *Annual Review of Nursing Research*, Springer, New York, pp183-208.

Cornett, J.W. (1995) The importance of systematic reflection: Implications of a naturalistic model of research, *Anthropology and Education Quarterly*, Vol. 26, No. 1, pp123-129.

Coser, L.A., Rosenberg, B. (1976) *Sociological Theory*, Fourth edition, Collier Macmillan International editions, Collier Macmillan Publishers, London.

Cowman, S. (1993) Triangulation: A means of reconciliation in nursing research, *Journal of Advanced Nursing*, Vol. 18, pp788-792.

Csordas, T.J. (ed) (1994) *Embodiment and Experience. The Existential Ground of Culture and Self.* Cambridge University Press.

Cull-Wilby, B.L. (1987) Towards a co-existence of paradigms in nursing knowledge development, *Journal of Advanced Nursing*, Vol. 12, pp515-521.

Davis, M.Z. (1986) Observation in natural settings, in Chenitz, W.C., Swanson, J.M. (eds), *From Practice to Grounded Theory*, Qualitative Research in Nursing, Addison Wesley, Wokingham, Berkshire.

Delamont, S. (1992) *Fieldwork in Educational Settings. Methods, Pitfalls and Perspectives*, The Falmer Press.

Denzin, N.K. (1970) *The Research Act*, Aldine Publishing Co, Chicago.

Denzin, N.K. (1977) *Childhood Socialization*, Jossey Bass, San Francisco.

Denzin, N.K. (1978) *Sociological Methods. A Sourcebook*, 2nd Edition. McGraw Hill, New York.

Denzin, N.K. (1989) *Interpretive Interactionism*, Newbury Park, Sage, CA.

Denzin, N.K., Lincoln, Y.S. (eds) (1994) *Handbook of Qualitative Research*, Sage Publications, London.

Department of Health (1994) C.N.O. Letter 94(5), *Clinical Supervision for the Nursing and Health Visitor Professionals*, HMSO, London.

Drew, N. (1989) The Interviewers Experience as Data in Phenomenological Research, *Western Journal of Nursing Research*, Vol. 11, pp431-439.

Dudley, M., Butterworth, T. (1994) The cost and some benefits of clinical supervision: An initial exploration, *Journal of Psychiatric Nursing Research*, Vol. 1, No. 2, pp34-46.

Dufrenne, M. (1973) *Phenomenology of Aesthetic Experience*, North Western University Press, Evanston.

Elkan, R., Robinson, J. (1993) Project 2000: The gap between theory and practice, *Nurse Education Today*, Vol. 13, pp295-298.

Elkan, R., Robinson, J. (1995) Project 2000: A review of published research, *Journal of Advanced Nursing*, Vol. 22, pp386-392.

Estabrooks, C.A., Field, P.A., Morse, J.M. (1994) Aggregating qualitative findings: An approach to theory development, *Qualitative Health Research*, Vol. 4, No. 4, Nov. pp503-511.

Esterling Levy, S.M. (1975) Personal constructs and existential a priori categories, *Journal of Phenomenological Psychology*, Vol. 5, pp369-388.

Farkas-Cameron, M. (1995) Clinical supervision in psychiatric nursing, *Journal of Psychosocial Nursing*, Vol. 33, pp31-37.

Farrington, A. (1993) Intuition and expert clinical practice in nursing, *British Journal of Nursing*, Vol. 2, No. 4, pp228-233.

Ford, D.H. (1987) *Humans as Self-Constructing Living Systems. A Developmental Perspective on Behaviour and Personality*, Lawrence Erlbaum Associates, Publishers, Hillsdale, New Jersey.

Forrest, D. (1989) The experience of caring, *Journal of Advanced Nursing*, Vol. 14, pp815-823.

Foucault, M. cited in Gordon, C. (ed) (1980) *Michel Foucault, Power and Knowledge: Selected Interviews and Other Writings*, 1972-1977, New York.

Fowler, J. (1996) The organisation of clinical supervision within the nursing profession. A review of the literature, *Journal of Advanced Nursing*, Vol. 23, pp471-478.

Fowler, J., Chevannes, M. (1998) Evaluating the efficiency of reflective practice within the context of clinical supervision, *Journal of Advanced Nursing*, Vol. 27, pp379-382.

Fransella, F., Bannister, D. (1977) *A Manual for Repertory Grid Technique*, Academic Press, Harcourt Brace Jovanovich Publishers.

French, P. (1989) *An Assessment of the Pre-Registration Preparation of Nurses as an Educational Experience*, Unpublished PhD Thesis, University of Durham.

Gadamer, H.G. (1987) Hermeneutics as practical philosophy, in Bayner, K, Bohman, J and McCarthy, T. (eds) *After Philosophy: End or Transformation?* MIT Press, Cambridge, Massachusetts, pp319-350.

Gaut, D.A. (Ed) (1992) *The Presence of Caring in Nursing*, National league for Nursing Press, Newcastle.

Geer, B. (ed) (1972) *Learning to Work*, Sage, Beverley Hills, California.

Gilligan, C. (1978) In a different voice: Women's conception of the self and of morality, *Harvard Educational Review*, Vol. 47, No. 4, pp481-517.

Graham, H. (1991) The concept of caring in feminist research: The case of domestic service, *Sociology*, Vol. 25, No. 1, pp61-78.

Graham, I. (1994) How do registered nurses think and experience nursing? A phenomenological investigation, *Journal of Clinical Nursing*, Vol. 3, pp235-242.

Guignon, C. (ed) (1996) *The Cambridge Companion to Heidegger*, Cambridge University Press.

Habermas, J. (1987) *The Theory of Communicative Action*, Vol. 2, Polity, Cambridge.

Hammersley, M., Atkinson, P. (1983) *Ethnography: Principles in Practice*, Tavistock, London.

Haralambos, M. (1985) *Sociology. Themes and Perspectives*, 2nd edition, Unwin, Hyman.

Hardiman, R.H. (1993) Teachers experiences of their role following the implementation of Project 2000: A qualitative approach, *Journal of Advanced Nursing*, 18, pp1023-1032.

Harding, S. (1983) Towards a reflexive feminist theory, *Women Politics*, Vol. 3, No. 4, pp27-42.

310

Hardy, L.K., Segatore, M., Edge, D.S., (1993) Illiteracy: Implications for nursing education, *Nurse Education Today*, Vol. 13, pp24-29.

Haugeland, J. (1993) Daseins Disclosedness, Chapter 1, in Dreyfuss, H.L. (ed) *Heidegger: A Critical Reader*, Blackwell, Oxford.

Heidegger, M. (1982) *The Basic Problems with Phenomenology*, Indiana University Press.

Heidegger, M. (1997) *Being and Time*, Translated by Macquarrie, J., Robinson, E. Blackwell, Oxford.

Hisrich, R.D., Peters, M.P. (1982) *Focus groups: An innovative marketing research technique*, Hospital and Health Services Administration, July/August, pp8-21.

Hofstadter, A. (1988) *Martin Heidegger. The Basic Problems with Phenomenology*, Indiana University Press, Bloomington and Indianapolis.

Holden, R.J. (1991) In defence of Cartesian dualism and the hermeneutic horizon, *Journal of Advanced Nursing*, Vol. 16, pp1375-1381.

Hospers, J. (1989) *An Introduction to Philosophical Analysis*, Revised edition, Routledge, London.

Houston, G. (1993) *Being and Belonging. Group Intergroup and Gestalt*, John Wiley and Sons.

Howard, R.J. (1982) *Three Faces of Hermeneutics*, University of California Press Ltd., London, England.

Hurley, B.A. (1988) Socialization for roles, in Hardy, M.E., Conway, H.E. (eds) *Role Theory: Perspectives for Health Professionals*, 2nd edition, Appleton and Lange Norwalk, Connecticut, pp73-110.

Husserl, E. (1970) *Logical Investigations*, Translated by Findley, J.N. Vol. 1, Hermeneutics Press, New York, p28.

Jennings, J.L. (1986) Husserl revisited: The forgotten distinction between psychology and phenomenology, *American Psychologist*, Vol. 41, No. 11, pp1231-1240.

Johns, C. (1993) Professional supervision, *Journal of Nursing Management*, Vol. 1, pp9-18.

Jones, C., Porter, R. (eds) (1994) *Reassessing Foucault. Power, Medicine and the Body*, Routledge, London and New York.

Jowett, S., Walton, I., Payne, S. (1991) *Project 2000 Research - Interim Papers 1 + 2*, National Foundation for Educational Research, Slough, London.

Jowett, S., Walton, I., Payne, S. (1992) *The Introduction of Project 2000. Interim Papers 3 + 4*, National Foundation for Educational Research, Slough, London.

Kegan, R. (1996) *The Evolving Self*, Harvard University Press, Cambridge, Massachusetts and London, England.

Kelly, G.A. (1991) *The Psychology of Personal Constructs*, Vol. 1, A Theory of Personality, Routledge.

Kiger, A.M. (1993) Accord and discord in students. Images of Nursing, *Journal of Nursing Education*. Vol. 32, No. 7, Sept., pp309-317.

Knaak, P. (1984) Phenomenological research, *Western Journal of Nursing Research*, Vol. 6, No. 1, pp107-114.

Kohak, E. (1978) Ideas and Experience: Edmund Husserls Project of Phenomenology, in *Ideas*, 1, University of Chicago Press, Chicago.

Korner, S. (1969) *What is Philosophy*? The Penguin Press, Allen Lane.

Kovach, C. (1991) (1) Reminiscence: Exploring the origins, processes and consequences, *Nursing Forum*, Vol. 26, No. 3, pp14-26.

Kovach, C. (1991) (2) Content analysis of the reminiscences of elderly females, *Research in Nursing and Health*, Vol. 14, pp287-295.

Kramer, M. (1974) *Reality Shock: Why Nurses Leave Nursing*, CV Mosby, St Louis.

Kretlow, F. (1990) A phenomenological view of illness, *Australian Journal of Advanced Nursing*, Vol. 7, No. 2, pp8-10.

Kvale, S. (1983) The qualitative research interview, *Journal of Phenomenological Psychology*, Vol. 1, No. 2, pp171-196.

La Capre, D. (1978) *A Preface to Sartre*, Methuen and Co. Ltd.

Langer, M.M. (1989) *Merleau-Ponty's Phenomenology of Perception. A Guide and Commentary*, Macmillan Press.

Leonard, A., Jowett, S. (1990) *Charting the Course: A Study of the Six ENB Pilot Schemes in Pre-Registration Nurse Education*, NFER, London.

Lewis, M. (1990) The development of intentionality and the role of consciousness, *Psychological Inquiry*, Vol. 1, No. 3, pp231-247.

Lyons, W. (1990) Intentionality and modern philosophical psychology, 1, The modern reduction of intentionality, *Philosophical Inquiry*, Vol. 3, No. 2, pp247-269.

Macleod Clark, J., Maben, J., Jones, K. (1996) *Project 2000 Perceptions of the Philosophy and Practice of Nursing*, The Nightingale Institute, Kings College, London, ENB, London.

Macleod, R.B. (1947) The phenomenological approach in social psychology, *Psychological Review*, Vol. 54, pp193-210.

Magee, B. (1987) *The Great Philosophers: An Introduction to Western Philosophy*, Oxford University Press, Oxford.

Mallin, S.B. (1979) *Merleau-Ponty's Philosophy*, Yale University Press, New Haven and London, p8.

Malpas, J. (1992) Analysis and hermeneutics, *Philosophy and Rhetoric*, Vol. 25, pp93-123.

Markus, H., Nurius, P. (1986) Possible selves, *American Psychologist*, Vol. 41, No. 9, Sept. pp954-969.

Marrow, E. (1997) Promoting reflective practice through structured clinical supervision, *Journal of Nursing Management*, Vol. 5, pp77-82.

Marsick, V.J. (1987) *Learning in the Workplace*, Croomhelm, Bechenham, Kent.

May, F.E., Champion, V., Austin, J.K. (1991) Public values and beliefs toward nursing as a career, *Journal of Nursing Education*, Vol. 30, No. 7, pp303-310.

May, R. (1969) *Love and Will*, Souvenir Press, London.

Mazindu, G.N. (1992) Using repertory grid research methodology in nurse education and practice, *Journal of Advanced Nursing*, Vol. 17, pp604-608.

Melia, K.M. (1981) *Student Nurses Accounts of Their Work and Training. A Qualitative Analysis*, Unpublished PhD Thesis, University of Edinburgh.

Melia, K.M. (1987) *Learning and Working. The Occupational Socialization of Nurses*, Tavistock Publications.

Mergendoller, J.R. (1981) *War Resistance and Moral Experience*, University Microfilms International.

Mergendoller, J.R. (1989) Good and ill will. Wartime as the context for the study of moral action. In; Packer and Addison, *Entering the Circle*, Chapter 4, pp119-140.

Merleau-Ponty, M. (1962) *The Phenomenology of Perception*, Routledge and Kegan-Paul, London.

Merton, R.K. (1957) *The Student Physician*, Harvard University Press, Cambridge, Mass.

Morse, J.M., Bottorff, J.L., Hutchinson, S. (1994) The phenomenology of comfort, *Journal of Advanced Nursing*, Vol. 20, pp189-195.

Mortimer, J.T., Simmons, R.G. (1978) Adult socialization, *Annual Review of Sociology*, 4, pp421-454.

Moustakas, C. (1994) *Phenomenological Research Methods*, Sage Publications Inc., London.

Mueller-Vollmer, K. (1985) *The Hermeneutic Reader*, Blackwells, UK.

Orr, J.G. (1990) Tradition Vs Project 2000. Something old, something new, *Nurse Education Today*, Vol. 10, pp58-62.

Outhwaite, W. (1994) *Habermas - A Critical Introduction*, Polity Press, Oxford.

Outhwaite, W. (1996) *The Habermas Reader*, Polity Press, Oxford.

Packer, M.J., Addison, R.B. (eds) (1989) *Entering the Circle. Hermeneutic Investigation in Psychology*, State University of New York Press.

Pettigrew, J. (1988) Doctoral dissertation. Texas Womens University, *A Phenomenological Study of the Nurses Presence with Persons Experiencing Suffering*, University Microfilms, No. 88 - 21422.

Rabinow, P., Sullivan, W. (eds) (1987) The interpretive turn, in *Interpretive Social Science. A Second Look*, University of California Press, Berkeley, pp1-32.

Rader, M. (ed) (1979) *A Modern Book of Aesthetics: An Anthropology*, Holt, Rinehart and Winston, New York.

Reason, P. (1988) *Human Inquiry in Action*, Sage Publications, London, pp1-17.

Richardson, L. (1990) *Writing Strategies - Reaching Diverse Audiences*, Sage Publications Inc., London.

Ricoeur, P. (1996) *The Hermeneutics of Action*, Edited by Richard Kearney, Sage Publications, London.

Rockmore, T. (1992) *On Heidegger's Nazism and Philosophy*, Harvester Wheatsheaf, London.

Ryan, D., Mc Haffie, H.E. (1990) The socialisation of nurses in clinical settings: A dual focus critique of a research study, *Nurse Education Today*, April, Vol. 10, No. 2, pp151-155.

Sartre, J.P. (1996) *Being and Nothingness*, Routledge, London.

Schon, D.A. (1987) *Educating the Reflective Practitioner*. Jossey-Bass Publishers, London.

Seed, A. (1991) *Becoming a Registered Nurse - The Student's Perspective*, Unpublished PhD.thesis, Leeds Polytechnic.

Simpson, I.H. (1979) *From Student to Nurse: A Longitudinal Study of Socialisation*, Cambridge University Press, New York.

Smith, P.A. (1992) *The Emotional Labour of Nursing: How Nurses Care*, MacMillan, Basingstoke.

Stevens, R. (ed) (1996) *Understanding Self*, The Open University, Sage Publications, London.

Taylor, B.J. (1994) *Being Human: Ordinariness in Nursing*, Churchill Livingstone, Melbourne.

Taylor, C. (1989) *Sources of the Self*, MA; Harvard University Press, Cambridge.

Thompson, J.B. (1981) *Critical Hermeneutics. A Study in the Thought of Paul Ricoeur and Jurgen Habermas*, Cambridge, London.

United Kingdom Central Council (1986) *Project 2000: A New Preparation for Practice*, UKCC, London.

Van Manen, M. (1990) *Researching Lived Experience*, T. Althouse, London, Ontario.

Warnke, G. (1987) *Gadamer: Hermeneutics, Tradition and Reason*, Polity Press, Cambridge.

Waterhouse, R. (1981) *A Heidegger Critique*, Harvester Press, Sussex.

White, E., Rliey, E., Davies, S., Twinn, S. (1993) *A Detailed Study of the Relationships Between Teaching, Support, Supervision and Role Modelling for Students in*

Clinical Areas Within the Context of Project 2000, Kings College London and University of Manchester, ENB.

Wilson-Barnett, J., Butterworth, T., White, E., Twinn, S., Davies, S., Riley, L. (1995) Clinical support and the Project 2000 nursing student: Factors influencing this process, *Journal of Advanced Nursing*, Vol. 21, pp1152-1158.

Woods, P. (1999) *Successful Writing for Qualitative Researchers*, Routledge, London and New York.